LEGS FOR DAYS: The Complete Hip & Thigh Workout BIBLE

Transform Your Lower Body with Power-Packed Routines for Strength, Shape, and Confidence

PETER COX

DEDICATION

To my family, whose unwavering support and love have been my foundation,

To my friends, who have inspired and encouraged me every step of the way,

And to all the dreamers and doers, who strive for success and never give up,

This book is dedicated to you.

May it be a guide and a source of inspiration on your journey to achieving your dreams.

With heartfelt gratitude.

Abstract

Legs for Days is the ultimate guide to building a strong, sculpted, and resilient lower body through expertly crafted workouts focused on the hips, thighs, and glutes. This comprehensive book provides a step-by-step approach to transforming your lower body, whether you're aiming for increased strength, improved shape, or enhanced overall fitness. It begins by demystifying the anatomy of the hips and thighs, allowing readers to understand the key muscle groups involved and how each contributes to stability, mobility, and lower body power. From foundational bodyweight moves to advanced strength and conditioning exercises, *Legs for Days* offers a range of routines suitable for beginners through advanced fitness enthusiasts.

In addition to exercises, the book dives into essential topics such as goal setting, tracking progress, and maintaining motivation to help readers stay committed to their fitness journeys. It also covers key lifestyle components, including nutrition and recovery, essential for supporting muscle growth and preventing injuries. With detailed instructions, workout plans, and form tips, *Legs for Days* empowers readers to build not only strength and endurance but also confidence and a positive relationship with their bodies.

Designed to be both inspirational and actionable, this book encourages readers to embrace the challenge and enjoy the rewards of a fitness journey that will not only shape their legs but also enhance their overall quality of life. Perfect for those looking to achieve lasting results and a lifetime of healthy movement, *Legs for Days* is the definitive guide to unlocking the strength, stability, and aesthetics of a powerful lower body.

TABLE OF CONTENT

The Importance of Lower Body Strength 8

Confidence Through Fitness 10

Overview of the Book 11

Part 1: Understanding Your Lower Body 15

Key Muscles: An Overview of the Major Muscle
Groups in the Hips, Thighs, and Glutes 15

Why Anatomy Matters in Your Fitness Journey 21

How These Muscles Work Together: Role of Each
Muscle in Movement, Strength, and Stability 22

Common Myths and Misconceptions: Debunking
Myths About Lower Body Transformation 27

Key Takeaways 33

Strength and Stability: How Training the Lower Body
Supports Balance, Posture, and Core Strength 35

Health and Longevity: The Role of Leg Strength in
Preventing Injuries, Improving Joint Health, and
Supporting Cardiovascular Fitness 41

Weight Loss and Fat Burning: The Impact of Lower
Body Workouts on Metabolism and Fat Loss 47

Chapter 3: Getting Started – Goal Setting and
Motivation 54

1. Focus on the Journey, Not Just the Destination 59

2. Set Micro-Goals and Celebrate Small Wins 60

3. Practice Positive Self-Talk and Visualization 60

4. Track Non-Scale Victories (NSVs) 61

5. Surround Yourself with Positive Influence 62

6. Learn to Appreciate Rest and Recovery 62

7. Accept Plateaus and Use Them as Learning Moments 63

Part 2: Power-Packed Lower Body Exercises .65

Chapter 4: Essential Hip and Thigh Exercises 65

Tips for Maximizing Bodyweight Exercises 72

Dumbbell and Kettlebell Variations: Adding Resistance for Strength, Growth, and Power 73

Tips for Maximizing Dumbbell and Kettlebell Workouts 81

Machine-Based Exercises: Targeted Strength and Isolation 82

Tips for Maximizing Machine-Based Exercises 89

Chapter 5: Glute-Focused Moves for Lift and Shape..90

Tips for Maximizing Glute Engagement 97

Tips for Perfect Form: Detailed Cues and Tips to Ensure Maximum Engagement and Prevent Common Mistakes 98

Importance of Glute Strength: How Stronger Glutes Improve Hip Alignment, Support Posture, and Reduce Lower Back Pain 101

Chapter 6: Inner and Outer Thigh Toning 104

Why Inner and Outer Thigh Strength Matters 111

Benefits of Toned Thighs: How Strengthening These Muscles Contributes to Overall Leg Shape and Stability 112

Resistance Band and Cable Machine Workouts: Using Bands and Cables to Add Intensity to Inner and Outer Thigh Exercises 116

Chapter 7: Core and Hip Flexor Activation 123

Preventing Tight Hip Flexors: Exercises and Stretches to Balance Hip Flexor Strength and Flexibility.........131

Part 3: Building Your Lower Body Routine ...136

Chapter 8: Designing Your Workout Plan 137

Chapter 9: Beginner Routines 142

Chapter 10: Intermediate Routines 147

Supersets and Circuits...151

Power and Performance-Based Training...................157

Targeted Workouts for Specific Goals.......................162

Part 4: Supporting Your Workouts with Nutrition and Lifestyle...166

Chapter 12: Nutrition for a Strong and Toned Lower Body 166

Chapter 13: Essential Stretches for Hips and Thighs 176

Benefits of Hip and Thigh Mobility Drills.................182

Chapter 14: Recovery Techniques and Injury Prevention..183

Sleep and Recovery: The Critical Role of Rest and Sleep in Muscle Repair, Energy Levels, and Fitness Progress..189

Part 5: Staying Motivated and Achieving Lasting Results...194

Chapter 15: Staying Consistent for Long-Term Success 194

Chapter 16: Building Confidence Through Fitness...202

Conclusion: Your Journey to Stronger, Sculpted Legs...217

Introduction: Why Strong, Toned Legs Matter

The journey to strong, toned legs is about more than just aesthetics—it's a path to building functional strength, improving mobility, and gaining confidence that radiates into every part of life. Our legs, particularly the hips and thighs, play a crucial role in our daily movements and overall physical health. In this introduction, we'll dive into the importance of building strength in the lower body, discuss how achieving toned legs can positively impact self-confidence, and provide an overview of what you can expect from this book.

The Importance of Lower Body Strength

Strong legs are the foundation of physical fitness and mobility. The muscles of the hips, thighs, and glutes support almost every move we make. Whether we're walking, running, lifting, or even standing, our legs bear much of the load. Building strength in the lower body improves stability, supports posture, and can even help prevent injuries. Here's a closer look at how lower body strength contributes to physical well-being:

- **Enhanced Mobility and Balance**: Strong hips, thighs, and glutes provide better stability and control, which helps with balance and coordination. This is especially important as we age, as muscle loss can lead to instability and a greater risk of falls. By strengthening these muscles, you can maintain better mobility and reduce the risk of accidents and injuries.

- **Support for Everyday Activities**: Many daily tasks—such as lifting heavy objects, climbing stairs, and even getting up from a seated position—require strength and stability from the legs. When these muscles are well-trained, everyday activities become easier and less strenuous. A strong lower body can relieve strain on the back and other areas of the body that might otherwise have to overcompensate for weak legs.

- **Increased Athletic Performance**: For those who enjoy sports or physical activities, a strong lower body is essential. Whether you're a runner, cyclist, dancer, or weekend athlete, the power in your hips and thighs fuels better performance. Strong legs help increase speed, endurance, and agility, allowing for a more dynamic range of movements and enhanced athletic performance.

- **Improved Metabolism and Fat Burning**: Lower body exercises, especially compound movements like squats and lunges, recruit multiple large muscle groups, which makes them more metabolically demanding. When these muscles are engaged and trained, they require a significant amount of energy, both during exercise and afterward as they recover. This increased energy expenditure helps boost metabolism and can aid in fat loss, which is particularly helpful for those aiming to shed excess body weight or tone up.

- **Joint Health and Injury Prevention**: Strengthening the legs, particularly the stabilizing muscles around the hips and knees, helps protect the joints. Many knee, hip, and back issues stem from weak or imbalanced leg muscles. By regularly training these muscles, you can improve joint stability, reduce stress on your knees and hips, and decrease the likelihood of injuries related to muscular imbalances.

Confidence Through Fitness

Achieving toned legs and a strong lower body can have a profound impact on self-confidence. When we feel strong and capable, it enhances not only how we feel physically but also how we view ourselves. Here's how developing lower body strength can positively affect confidence and body image:

- **Enhanced Self-Image**: Toned, sculpted legs are often seen as a hallmark of fitness, and working toward them can improve self-esteem and body positivity. Many people find that as they begin to see physical changes in their body—such as increased definition in the legs and glutes—they feel a greater sense of accomplishment. This progress, both visually and in how their body performs, can shift their relationship with their body to one of pride and appreciation.

- **Empowerment Through Strength**: There's a unique empowerment that comes from feeling physically strong. Lower body workouts, particularly those that involve weight lifting or resistance exercises, foster a sense of power and resilience. As strength improves, so does the ability to take on physical challenges that may have previously seemed difficult. This sense of capability often translates beyond the gym, instilling confidence that can be applied to other aspects of life.
- **Stress Relief and Mental Well-Being**: Exercise, including strength training, releases endorphins—natural chemicals that improve mood and alleviate stress. Working on lower body strength is not just a physical challenge; it's also a mental one that requires focus, determination, and patience. As you meet these challenges head-on, you may find a new sense of inner calm and satisfaction. Additionally, seeing physical progress can bring a sense of joy, reducing stress and boosting overall mental well-being.

Overview of the Book

This book is structured to be your complete guide to building strong, toned hips, thighs, and glutes. Divided into six parts, it provides a clear, progressive pathway to achieving your lower body goals. Here's a breakdown of what you'll find in each part:

1. **Understanding Your Lower Body**: The first section introduces the anatomy of the lower body, focusing on the major muscle groups in the hips, thighs, and glutes. This part also covers the benefits of lower body strength, common misconceptions, and how these muscles work together in various movements. This foundational knowledge sets the stage for the workouts to come.

2. **Power-Packed Lower Body Exercises**: In Part 2, you'll learn about essential exercises for targeting each area of the hips, thighs, and glutes. These exercises range from bodyweight basics to more advanced moves with weights and resistance bands, ensuring that readers of all fitness levels can find exercises suited to their needs. Each exercise includes form tips and variations to maximize effectiveness and prevent injury.

3. **Building Your Lower Body Routine**: Part 3 guides you through designing a workout routine tailored to your fitness level and goals. It includes beginner, intermediate, and advanced routines that progressively build strength, endurance, and muscle tone. You'll also learn about

important aspects like rep and set structures, rest, and recovery to optimize results.

4. **Supporting Your Workouts with Nutrition and Lifestyle**: Proper nutrition and recovery are critical for muscle growth and overall well-being. Part 4 provides advice on meal planning, nutrient timing, and essential recovery techniques like stretching and foam rolling to keep your body feeling and performing its best.

5. **Staying Motivated and Achieving Lasting Results**: Staying consistent with any fitness journey is often the biggest challenge. Part 5 offers practical tips and motivational strategies to help you overcome plateaus, celebrate small wins, and build a positive relationship with fitness and body image.

6. **Bringing It All Together**: The book concludes with a roadmap to long-term success, encouraging readers to embrace their fitness journey, celebrate their progress, and integrate lower body workouts into their lifestyle.

By following the routines and guidance in Legs for Days: The Complete Hip & Thigh Workout Bible, you will build strength, improve mobility, and gain confidence in your physical abilities. The comprehensive nature of this book ensures that you have the tools, knowledge, and motivation needed to achieve toned legs and a strong, stable lower body. Whether you're a beginner just getting started or an experienced fitness enthusiast seeking to up your game, this book is designed to be a go-to resource for sculpting your hips, thighs, and glutes.

Part 1: Understanding Your Lower Body

Chapter 1: Anatomy of the Hips and Thighs

Understanding the anatomy of the hips and thighs is essential to maximizing the effectiveness of your workouts and achieving a balanced, strong lower body. This chapter provides an overview of the key muscles in the hips, thighs, and glutes, which are vital for movement, stability, and strength. Knowing how these muscles function and work together will help you perform exercises with proper form, target specific areas more effectively, and reduce the risk of injury.

Key Muscles: An Overview of the Major Muscle Groups in the Hips, Thighs, and Glutes

The hips, thighs, and glutes are home to some of the body's most powerful and functional muscles. These muscles are responsible for movement, stabilization, and supporting the weight of the upper body. Here's a breakdown of each major muscle group:

1. Quadriceps (Front of the Thigh)

The quadriceps, often called "quads," are a group of four muscles located at the front of the thigh. These muscles are among the largest in the body and are primarily responsible for extending (straightening) the knee. Strong quads are essential for movements like walking, running, squatting, and jumping.

- **Muscles in the Quadriceps Group**: The four muscles of the quadriceps include the rectus femoris, vastus lateralis, vastus medialis, and vastus intermedius.
- **Function and Importance**: The quads play a significant role in knee stabilization and contribute to power generation for explosive movements, like sprinting or jumping. Having strong quads can improve athletic performance and protect the knee joint from injuries.

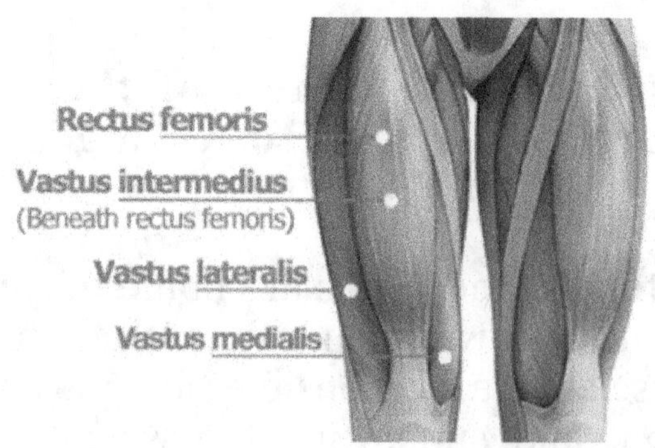

2. Hamstrings (Back of the Thigh)

The hamstrings are a group of three muscles located at the back of the thigh. These muscles work opposite the quadriceps, allowing the knee to bend (flex) and the hip to extend (move backward). The hamstrings are crucial for movements that require hip extension and knee flexion, such as running, deadlifting, and climbing stairs.

- **Muscles in the Hamstrings Group**: The hamstrings consist of the biceps femoris, semitendinosus, and semimembranosus.
- **Function and Importance**: Strong hamstrings help stabilize the pelvis, support the hips, and prevent imbalances that can lead to knee and lower back injuries. They are also key for explosive power and speed in athletic activities.

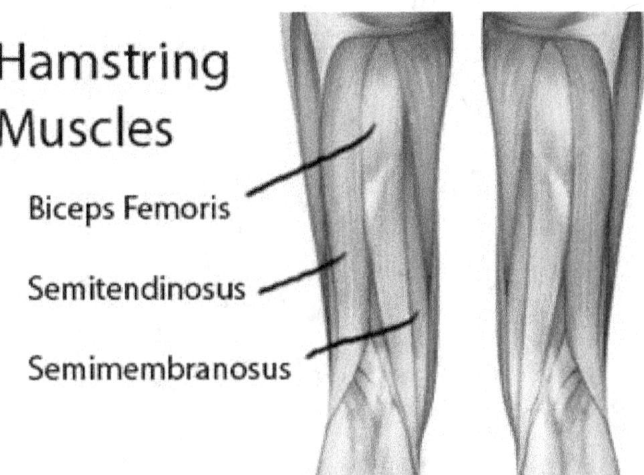

3. Adductors (Inner Thigh)

The adductor muscles are located along the inner thigh and are responsible for bringing the legs toward the midline of the body (adduction). These muscles play an important role in stabilizing the hips and pelvis, especially during lateral movements and exercises that require balance.

- **Muscles in the Adductor Group**: The adductor group includes the adductor longus, adductor brevis, adductor magnus, gracilis, and pectineus.
- **Function and Importance**: Strong adductors help stabilize the pelvis, improve balance, and aid in lower body movements like side lunges or any exercises involving lateral motion. Strengthening these muscles can also enhance athletic performance, particularly in sports that require quick changes in direction.

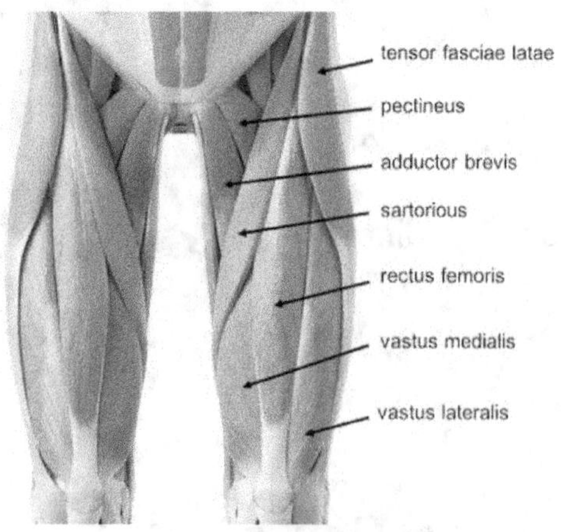

4. Gluteal Muscles (Buttocks)

The gluteal muscles, commonly known as the glutes, are located in the buttocks and are one of the body's most powerful muscle groups. They consist of three main muscles that play a central role in stabilizing the pelvis, extending the hip, and supporting a wide range of lower body movements.

- **Muscles in the Gluteal Group**: The three main muscles in this group are the gluteus maximus, gluteus medius, and gluteus minimus.
    - **Gluteus Maximus**: The largest muscle in the gluteal group and one of the strongest in the body, the gluteus maximus is responsible for hip extension and outward rotation of the hip. It's activated in exercises like squats, lunges, and hip thrusts.
    - **Gluteus Medius and Minimus**: These smaller muscles are located on the outer hip and play a vital role in stabilizing the pelvis and supporting lateral movements. They're engaged in movements like side lunges, lateral band walks, and hip abductions.
- **Function and Importance**: The glutes are integral to nearly all lower body movements and play a key role in posture, balance, and injury prevention. Strong glutes can help alleviate lower back pain, support the knees, and enhance athletic performance by improving explosiveness and stability.

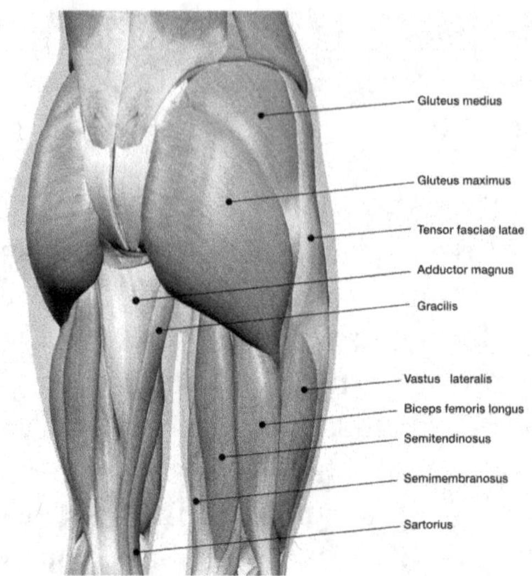

How These Muscle Groups Work Together

The muscles in the hips, thighs, and glutes do not work in isolation; they operate together in a coordinated fashion during lower body movements. For example:

- **Squats**: The quads, hamstrings, glutes, and adductors work together to lower and lift the body, providing power and stability.
- **Lunges**: The quads, hamstrings, and glutes are heavily engaged, while the adductors and abductors assist in maintaining balance.
- **Deadlifts**: This movement activates the hamstrings and glutes, with the quads and adductors providing additional support and stabilization.

Understanding this synergy is crucial for selecting exercises that effectively target each muscle group while avoiding imbalances.

Why Anatomy Matters in Your Fitness Journey

Knowing the anatomy of your hips and thighs isn't just for academic knowledge—it has practical applications that can directly improve your workouts:

- **Enhanced Exercise Form and Technique**: With a basic understanding of muscle groups and how they function, you'll be able to perform exercises with better form, targeting specific muscles more effectively and reducing strain on joints and surrounding muscles.
- **Efficient Targeting and Development**: Once you know which muscles you're working on, you can be intentional in your exercise selection and focus on areas that may need extra attention. For example, if you find your glutes or adductors are weaker, you can include additional exercises to strengthen them and build balanced lower body strength.
- **Injury Prevention**: Weak or underdeveloped muscles can lead to compensations elsewhere in the body, increasing the risk of strains and injuries. By understanding and strengthening all the major muscles in the lower body, you can

create a balanced, functional foundation that helps prevent injuries and supports overall body alignment.

How These Muscles Work Together: Role of Each Muscle in Movement, Strength, and Stability

The muscles of the hips, thighs, and glutes don't work in isolation—they function as a coordinated system to provide movement, strength, and stability in nearly every lower body exercise and daily activity. Understanding how each muscle works in concert with the others is key to optimizing your workouts, improving posture, and preventing injury. Here's how these muscles collaborate:

---

1. Quadriceps: Power and Extension

The **quadriceps** are primarily responsible for extending the knee joint, which is essential for movements such as standing up from a seated position, walking, squatting, and running.

- **Role in Movement**: During exercises like squats, lunges, and leg presses, the quads are the primary muscles that straighten the knee and extend the leg. When standing or walking, the quadriceps help propel the body forward by straightening the knee and stabilizing the lower leg.

- **Role in Strength**: The quadriceps are crucial for generating strength during lower body movements. The more powerful your quads are, the more weight you can handle in exercises like squats or leg presses, and the more explosive your movement can be in sports.
- **Role in Stability**: While the quads are responsible for moving the knee joint, they also work in synergy with the hamstrings and glutes to stabilize the knee during dynamic movements. When the quads contract to extend the leg, the hamstrings and glutes contract to balance the movement and control the knee's stability, preventing hyperextension.

---

2. Hamstrings: Flexion and Stabilization

The **hamstrings** are responsible for bending the knee and extending the hip. They are the antagonist muscles to the quadriceps, meaning they counteract the quads during movements and help stabilize the body during lower body activities.

- **Role in Movement**: In movements like deadlifts, running, and lunges, the hamstrings contract to flex the knee and extend the hip. For example, in a **deadlift**, as you hinge at the hips and lower the barbell, the hamstrings lengthen, and as you stand back up, they contract to extend the hips and straighten the body.

- **Role in Strength**: The hamstrings help provide balance and prevent overuse injuries to the quads. Strong hamstrings contribute to athletic performance by enabling quick acceleration, deceleration, and changes in direction. A well-developed hamstring also supports the lower back and prevents lower back strain during lifting and bending activities.
- **Role in Stability**: The hamstrings act as stabilizers by helping to control knee movement during exercises. They prevent the knee from overextending during squats and lunges, working in harmony with the quads to maintain proper knee alignment and reduce the risk of injury.

3. Adductors: Stability and Control

The **adductors** are a group of muscles along the inner thigh responsible for bringing the legs toward the body's midline (adduction). These muscles stabilize the pelvis and play a key role in controlling lateral movements.

- **Role in Movement**: During side lunges, lateral leg raises, or any movement involving crossing the legs over the midline, the adductors are actively engaged. They stabilize the pelvis and maintain balance while you move the legs in various directions, like in lateral walking or side-to-side steps.

- **Role in Strength**: Adductors provide additional power in activities that require leg movement across the body's midline, such as martial arts, dancing, or sports that involve cutting and direction changes. Strong adductors support a solid base of lower body strength, which helps with balance and coordination.
- **Role in Stability**: The adductors help stabilize the pelvis and support the spine, especially during squats or deadlifts. They assist in keeping the hips level during exercises, preventing the pelvis from tilting or shifting too much, which ensures that the movement is performed in a controlled manner.

4. Glutes: Power and Stability

The **glutes** (gluteus maximus, medius, and minimus) are the powerhouse muscles of the lower body and play a vital role in hip extension, stabilization, and movement. The glutes are responsible for providing the power needed for many lower body exercises and movements.

- **Role in Movement**: During movements like squats, lunges, and hip thrusts, the glutes are responsible for extending the hips and pushing the body upward. In actions like running, the glutes also assist in propelling the body forward with each stride. They stabilize the hips and legs, which is especially important when you are changing direction or lifting heavy weights.

- **Role in Strength**: Strong glutes are essential for producing power and explosive movement. They are involved in nearly every lower body exercise, especially compound lifts like squats, deadlifts, and lunges. The glutes also contribute to core stability and overall body strength, which is crucial for athletic performance.
- **Role in Stability**: The glutes, particularly the **gluteus medius**, play a significant role in stabilizing the pelvis and maintaining proper alignment. During single-leg exercises (like lunges or step-ups), the glutes prevent the pelvis from tilting or dropping on the opposite side. They also help with posture by keeping the spine aligned and preventing excessive arching or rounding of the back.

5. How These Muscle Groups Work Together

In any lower body exercise, the quadriceps, hamstrings, adductors, and glutes are working in unison to create smooth, coordinated movement. For example:

- **Squats**: As you lower your body into a squat, the **quadriceps** extend the knees while the **hamstrings** and **glutes** engage to control the descent. The **adductors** help keep the legs in alignment and prevent the knees from caving inwards.
- **Lunges**: When performing lunges, the **glutes** and **quads** are the primary movers, extending the hip and knee as you step forward. The **hamstrings** and **adductors** provide stability and support for the knees and hips, preventing strain or overextension.
- **Running**: The **quadriceps** extend the knee with each stride, while the **hamstrings** and **glutes** work to propel the body forward and provide thrust. The **adductors** stabilize the legs during the push-off phase to ensure a smooth, balanced stride.

Common Myths and Misconceptions: Debunking Myths About Lower Body Transformation

The fitness world is filled with myths and misconceptions, especially when it comes to achieving toned, strong hips and thighs. These myths can often lead to frustration or confusion, leaving people feeling discouraged when they don't see the results they expect. It's important to address these myths so that you can approach your lower body transformation with realistic expectations and an informed mindset. Let's take a closer look at some of the most common myths:

---

1. Spot Reduction: You Can Lose Fat in Specific Areas

Myth: Performing exercises that target specific areas of the body, such as squats or lunges for the thighs, will reduce fat specifically in that area (like "spot reducing" thigh fat).

Reality: Spot reduction is a myth. While exercises like squats, lunges, and leg presses can tone and strengthen the muscles in your hips, thighs, and glutes, they will not directly reduce fat in those areas. Fat loss occurs through a combination of overall body fat reduction (via diet and cardio) and strength training. You cannot choose where you lose fat; it's determined by genetics and overall body composition.

To reduce fat in the lower body (or anywhere else), you need to focus on overall fat loss through a healthy, balanced diet, regular cardiovascular exercise, and full-body strength training. As you reduce overall body fat, you'll see a slimmer, leaner appearance in all areas of the body, including the legs.

---

2. Heavy Weightlifting Will Make Your Legs Look Bulky

Myth: Lifting heavy weights, especially for the legs, will cause the thighs and hips to become bulky and oversized.

Reality: While heavy weightlifting can lead to muscle growth, it's highly unlikely to make your legs look overly bulky unless you're following a specialized program designed to build muscle mass significantly (such as bodybuilding) and consuming a surplus of calories for muscle growth.

For most people, lifting heavy weights will create lean, sculpted muscles that increase strength and definition without causing excessive bulk. Women, in particular, often fear "bulking up" due to lower testosterone levels, which means that building bulky muscle is much harder for women than men. Instead, lifting heavy weights will help you build strength and muscle tone, giving your legs a more athletic, sculpted look.

3. You Need to Do Endless Cardio to Lose Leg Fat

Myth: Cardio is the best or only way to burn fat and achieve toned legs.

Reality: While cardio does play a role in fat loss, it is not the only or the most effective way to achieve toned legs. In fact, a combination of **strength training** and **cardiovascular exercise** will yield the best results. Strength training helps build muscle, which boosts metabolism and helps you burn more calories even at rest. Additionally, muscle tissue burns more calories than fat tissue, meaning that as you build muscle in your legs, you'll help promote fat loss across your entire body.

A well-rounded fitness program that combines both cardio (such as walking, running, or cycling) with strength training (focusing on exercises like squats, lunges, and leg presses) is the most effective approach for achieving lean, strong, and toned legs.

4. You Can't Tone or Sculpt Your Legs Without Losing Weight

Myth: Toning your thighs and hips requires weight loss first, and you can't make any significant changes to these areas until you lose fat.

Reality: While losing fat will certainly help reveal toned muscles, you can still build muscle and improve the appearance of your legs regardless of your current weight. Strength training exercises like squats, lunges, and deadlifts will build muscle and give your legs shape and definition, whether you're losing fat or not.

That being said, a combination of muscle-building exercises and fat-burning cardio will give you the best chance to see a leaner, more sculpted appearance over time. But don't get discouraged—muscle tone and strength can be achieved even if fat loss is not the primary goal.

---

5. You Have to Work Out Your Legs Every Day to See Results

Myth: To get toned, strong legs, you need to work out your lower body every single day.

Reality: Overworking your legs is not only unnecessary, but it can also lead to burnout or injury. Muscles need time to recover in order to grow and become stronger. In fact, working out the same muscles every day without adequate rest can lead to overtraining, which can result in decreased performance, fatigue, and even injury.

For optimal results, it's important to give your lower body muscles time to recover between workouts. Aim for 2-3 strength training sessions per week for your lower body, with rest days in between to allow your muscles to recover. On non-strength training days, you can incorporate low-impact cardio or rest to avoid overexertion.

6. Leg Workouts Only Target Your Legs

Myth: Lower body exercises like squats and lunges only work the legs.

Reality: While leg-focused exercises do target the hips, thighs, and glutes, they also engage a variety of other muscles in the body. **Squats**, for example, work your core muscles, lower back, and even your upper body as you stabilize the movement. **Lunges** activate your core to maintain balance, and exercises like **deadlifts** engage your hamstrings, glutes, and lower back while also activating your forearms and grip strength.

Incorporating full-body movements into your lower body routine helps to improve overall strength and coordination while maximizing calorie burn. Strengthening your core and upper body alongside your legs is key to achieving a well-balanced and toned physique.

7. Stretching Is All You Need to Tone Legs

Myth: Stretching is enough to shape and tone your legs. You don't need strength exercises.

Reality: While stretching is important for flexibility and injury prevention, it is not sufficient on its own to tone or sculpt your legs. To build strength, muscle, and definition in your thighs, hips, and glutes, strength training is essential. Stretching can help improve your range of motion and reduce tightness, but it does not provide the resistance needed to stimulate muscle growth and fat loss.

Incorporate a combination of strength training exercises with stretching to achieve a toned, balanced lower body. Stretching should be part of your cool-down routine to help your muscles recover and prevent stiffness.

Key Takeaways

- **Spot reduction** doesn't work; fat loss occurs throughout the body, not in specific areas.
- **Heavy weightlifting** won't make your legs bulky unless you're deliberately training for mass.
- **Cardio** should be combined with strength training for the best results.
- **Rest** is crucial for muscle recovery and growth—don't overtrain.
- **Leg workouts** engage multiple muscle groups, providing full-body benefits.
- **Stretching** is important, but it's strength training that builds toned, strong legs.

By understanding and debunking these common myths, you can set more realistic and effective goals for your lower body transformation. Focus on a balanced approach that includes both strength training and cardio, and remember that transformation takes time. Consistency, patience, and a positive mindset are the key ingredients for success.

Chapter 2: The Benefits of Hip and Thigh Workouts

Strength and Stability: How Training the Lower Body Supports Balance, Posture, and Core Strength

The hips and thighs are among the most powerful areas of the body, forming the foundation for nearly every movement, from walking and running to bending and lifting. When you train these areas, you're not only working toward stronger and more toned legs but also enhancing your overall strength, stability, and posture. Understanding the benefits of hip and thigh workouts will help you appreciate how essential lower body training is for functional fitness and injury prevention. Let's explore the powerful ways these workouts contribute to balance, posture, and core strength.

---

1. Strength and Stability in Everyday Movements

The muscles in the hips, thighs, and glutes (collectively known as the lower body) are involved in nearly every movement you make. Whether you're standing up from a seated position, climbing stairs, or simply walking, these muscles play a central role. Training the lower body not only increases the strength of these muscles but also enhances their endurance and stability, making everyday movements easier and more efficient. Strong hips and thighs provide a solid base that helps prevent wobbly, unsteady movements, reducing the risk of trips and falls, especially as we age.

- **Examples of Strength-Building Exercises**: Exercises like squats, lunges, and deadlifts are ideal for building strength in the hips and thighs. They also activate stabilizing muscles in the legs and core, improving stability for both dynamic movements (like running) and static positions (like balancing on one foot).

2. Improved Balance and Coordination

Lower body strength is essential for balance and coordination. When you strengthen your hips, thighs, and glutes, you are better able to maintain control over your movements, which is critical for stability in various activities. The hip muscles, including the gluteus medius and gluteus minimus, are especially important for lateral stability—keeping you steady when moving side-to-side or shifting weight from one leg to the other.

Enhanced balance and coordination mean you're less likely to stumble or fall, which is particularly beneficial for older adults. But it also has advantages in athletics and other physical activities that require quick directional changes and agility. For example, sports like tennis, basketball, and skiing demand rapid, controlled movements that rely on strong, balanced lower body muscles.

- **Balance-Boosting Exercises**: Single-leg exercises, like single-leg deadlifts or lunges, help train balance by forcing you to stabilize through one leg. These moves also improve proprioception (your body's ability to sense where it is in space), which is key to coordination.

3. Enhanced Posture and Alignment

Good posture isn't just about having a strong back—it also relies on strong hips and thighs. The glutes and hip flexors work in tandem to stabilize the pelvis, which is the foundation of your spinal alignment. When these muscles are weak, it can lead to poor posture and imbalances that place unnecessary strain on the lower back.

By strengthening the hip flexors, glutes, and thigh muscles, you help to create a balanced posture that distributes weight evenly across the body. This reduces the risk of back pain and discomfort and encourages a more upright stance. Lower body strength training also combats the effects of prolonged sitting, which often causes tight hip flexors and weak glutes, leading to postural issues like anterior pelvic tilt (where the pelvis tilts forward, causing a swayback posture).

- **Posture-Improving Exercises**: Glute bridges, hip thrusts, and hip flexor stretches help open up tight hip flexors and activate the glutes, aligning the pelvis for better posture.

---

4. Core Strength and Stability

A strong lower body is closely tied to core strength, as the hips and thighs are integral to core stability. Your core isn't just your abs—it's the entire area that includes your pelvis, lower back, and glutes. When you perform lower body exercises like squats and lunges, your core has to engage to keep your body balanced and aligned.

This engagement strengthens the core muscles and improves their ability to stabilize the spine, which is crucial for preventing lower back injuries. Core stability also allows for efficient power transfer between the upper and lower body, making movements more fluid and efficient, whether you're lifting weights, playing sports, or simply moving throughout your day.

- **Core-Stabilizing Lower Body Exercises**: Compound exercises like deadlifts, squats, and Bulgarian split squats require core stabilization to perform correctly, promoting both core strength and stability as you train your lower body.

5. Injury Prevention and Joint Protection

Weak hips and thighs can lead to imbalances that increase the risk of injuries, particularly in the knees, lower back, and hips. For example, weak glutes can cause the knees to cave inward during activities like squatting or running, putting strain on the knee joint. By strengthening the muscles around the hips and thighs, you're creating a protective "armor" for these joints, helping to prevent common issues like runner's knee, IT band syndrome, and hip impingement.

Additionally, lower body exercises help reinforce the ligaments and tendons in the knees, hips, and ankles. These connective tissues play a crucial role in stabilizing the joints, and regular lower body strength training can enhance their resilience, reducing the risk of strains, sprains, and other soft tissue injuries.

- **Injury-Preventing Exercises**: Exercises that engage the gluteus medius, such as side lunges and clamshells, strengthen the outer hip muscles, which are crucial for knee alignment and joint protection.

6. Power and Performance in Physical Activities

For athletes and active individuals, lower body strength is essential for peak performance. Strong hips, thighs, and glutes provide the explosive power needed for activities that involve jumping, sprinting, or lifting. Lower body workouts that focus on strength and plyometric exercises (like box jumps and explosive lunges) train the fast-twitch muscle fibers, which are responsible for quick bursts of power.

Enhanced lower body power doesn't just benefit competitive athletes; it's also valuable for recreational activities and hobbies, from hiking and cycling to dancing and swimming. Training these muscles ensures you have the strength and endurance needed for your favorite activities, allowing you to enjoy them safely and with less fatigue.

- **Performance-Enhancing Exercises**: Plyometric exercises like jump squats, box jumps, and kettlebell swings help build explosive power in the hips and thighs, which can enhance athletic performance.

Training your hips and thighs is about more than just achieving a toned, aesthetic look. It plays a fundamental role in strengthening your entire body, improving stability, posture, and core strength, as well as protecting against injuries. By prioritizing lower body strength and incorporating a range of exercises, you can build a foundation of strength and stability that will benefit every aspect of your life—from daily tasks to high-intensity sports.

This book will guide you through targeted exercises, form tips, and routines that focus on building strength, balance, and endurance in the hips and thighs. With a strong, resilient lower body, you'll feel more confident, empowered, and capable of tackling any physical challenge. Let's get started on transforming your lower body and enhancing your overall fitness with workouts that truly make a difference!

Health and Longevity: The Role of Leg Strength in Preventing Injuries, Improving Joint Health, and Supporting Cardiovascular Fitness

Strengthening your legs isn't just about building muscle or achieving a toned appearance; it plays a significant role in promoting long-term health, preventing injuries, and supporting overall longevity. Strong, healthy legs contribute to better joint function, reduce the risk of age-related injuries, and even enhance cardiovascular health. This foundational strength supports movement and independence well into later life, empowering people to stay active and engaged as they age. Below, we'll dive into the vital role that leg strength plays in injury prevention, joint health, and cardiovascular fitness.

---

1. Injury Prevention and Reduced Fall Risk

Maintaining strong leg muscles, especially in the hips, thighs, and glutes, significantly lowers the risk of injuries such as strains, sprains, and fractures. Falls are a major cause of injury among older adults, but strong legs help improve balance, coordination, and stability, which are critical for preventing these accidents. By regularly working on leg strength, you create a solid foundation that enhances control over your movements, especially during dynamic or quick shifts in position.

Strengthening the lower body also mitigates the risk of acute and overuse injuries. For example, muscles around the knee, such as the quadriceps and hamstrings, provide structural support and stability, which protects the joint during activities like running or jumping. Additionally, exercises that target the glutes help maintain proper alignment of the hips and knees, which reduces stress on the joints and ligaments, further lowering injury risk.

- **Exercises for Injury Prevention**: Movements such as squats, lunges, and single-leg exercises (e.g., single-leg deadlifts or balance work) enhance stability and control while training the muscles that protect and stabilize the joints.

2. Improving Joint Health and Mobility

Joint health often declines with age, leading to conditions like arthritis, which can limit mobility and cause discomfort. However, regular leg training can help improve joint health and prevent degeneration. Building strength around the joints provides extra stability, relieving pressure on the joints themselves. Strong muscles and tendons around the knees, hips, and ankles act as "shock absorbers," distributing force during movement, which reduces wear and tear on the joints over time.

Strengthening exercises also help maintain a full range of motion and flexibility, which supports joint function and prevents stiffness. Leg exercises that involve both concentric (muscle shortening) and eccentric (muscle lengthening) actions are particularly beneficial for the joints, as they stimulate the connective tissues, making them stronger and more resilient. For example, the controlled lowering phase in a squat enhances knee joint stability while working the surrounding muscles.

- **Joint Health-Boosting Exercises**: Low-impact movements like leg presses, hip bridges, and resistance band exercises target joint-supporting muscles without putting excessive stress on the joints themselves.

---

3. Supporting Cardiovascular Fitness

Many leg workouts, especially those involving large muscle groups, have cardiovascular benefits. Training the legs requires significant energy, which stimulates the cardiovascular system and promotes heart health. Exercises like squats, lunges, and cycling engage the large muscles in the lower body, increasing your heart rate and improving blood circulation. Regular leg training also enhances the efficiency of the cardiovascular system, as it learns to supply blood and oxygen more effectively to the working muscles.

Cardiovascular benefits from leg training go beyond short-term fitness improvements. Studies have shown that lower body strength is closely linked with reduced mortality rates, as well as a lower risk of heart disease and other chronic conditions. Engaging in consistent lower body workouts can improve cardiovascular endurance, which is critical for overall health and longevity.

- **Cardio-Strength Exercises for Leg Fitness**: Exercises like jump squats, step-ups, and kettlebell swings provide both strength and cardiovascular benefits, promoting a healthy heart while building leg strength.

4. Longevity and Quality of Life

Lower body strength is a powerful predictor of overall longevity and quality of life. As people age, maintaining leg strength can prevent the loss of independence by enabling basic mobility functions such as getting out of a chair, climbing stairs, and walking unassisted. Leg strength and balance are directly related to maintaining functional mobility, and a strong lower body can help people retain their independence well into their later years.

Moreover, preserving muscle mass in the legs combats sarcopenia (age-related muscle loss), which is a common issue as people age. Sarcopenia not only limits physical capabilities but also impacts metabolic health. Strong leg muscles contribute to metabolic efficiency, which helps regulate body weight, blood sugar, and energy levels. Leg strength is also associated with cognitive benefits, as regular exercise promotes blood flow to the brain, which supports mental clarity and cognitive health over time.

- **Exercises for Longevity and Functional Strength**: Compound movements like deadlifts, lunges, and leg presses are ideal for building functional strength, promoting longevity by preparing the body for the demands of daily life.

5. Boosting Metabolism and Supporting Weight Management

Strong leg muscles contribute to a higher resting metabolic rate, as muscle tissue burns more calories than fat, even at rest. Building and maintaining leg muscle mass, therefore, plays an essential role in supporting a healthy metabolism and managing body weight. This can be particularly beneficial for those aiming to lose weight or prevent age-related weight gain, as lower body training contributes to total body calorie burn.

Leg exercises that involve multiple joints and large muscle groups are particularly effective at maximizing calorie expenditure, even hours after a workout. High-intensity leg workouts, such as circuit-style training or plyometrics, can also promote a phenomenon known as excess post-exercise oxygen consumption (EPOC), where the body continues to burn calories after exercise as it returns to its resting state.

- **Metabolism-Boosting Leg Exercises**: High-intensity interval training (HIIT) exercises, like jump lunges, burpees, and squat jumps, provide an efficient way to boost metabolism and burn calories while strengthening the legs.

Strong, toned legs are more than a fitness goal—they are key to health, longevity, and a better quality of life. Building leg strength protects the joints, aids in injury prevention, supports cardiovascular fitness, and enhances metabolic health. As you train your lower body, you're investing in the durability and functionality of your body, ensuring you can continue to move, play, and engage in activities you love throughout your life.

With this book's workouts and techniques, you'll be equipped to maximize your lower body's potential, achieving greater strength, resilience, and wellness for years to come.

Weight Loss and Fat Burning: The Impact of Lower Body Workouts on Metabolism and Fat Loss

Lower body workouts are a powerful tool for weight loss and fat burning. Engaging the muscles in the hips, thighs, and glutes not only strengthens and tones but also significantly boosts metabolism, making it easier to shed excess body fat. Because these muscle groups are some of the largest in the body, targeting them results in a higher calorie burn both during and after workouts, thanks to the energy demands required by these powerful muscles.

Here's a closer look at how lower body workouts impact metabolism, promote fat loss, and support sustainable weight management.

1. Increased Calorie Burn with Lower Body Workouts

Training the lower body with compound exercises (those involving multiple joints and muscles) requires a lot of energy, making it one of the most effective ways to burn calories. Exercises like squats, lunges, and deadlifts use large muscles such as the quadriceps, hamstrings, and glutes, which naturally burn more calories compared to smaller muscles. The higher the intensity and complexity of the movement, the greater the calorie expenditure.

When performed at moderate to high intensity, lower body exercises can significantly boost your overall calorie burn, which is essential for fat loss. For example, high-rep, high-weight squats or lunges can increase your heart rate and challenge your body, leading to a caloric deficit essential for weight loss.

- **Calorie-Burning Lower Body Exercises**: Try incorporating compound movements like barbell squats, kettlebell swings, and walking lunges to maximize calorie burn and keep your heart rate elevated throughout the workout.

2. Metabolism Boost through Muscle Growth

One of the major benefits of lower body training is its impact on metabolism. Muscle tissue is metabolically active, meaning it burns more calories at rest than fat tissue. Therefore, by building and maintaining leg muscle, you can raise your basal metabolic rate (BMR)—the number of calories your body needs to function at rest. This is a crucial factor in weight loss and maintaining a lean body composition over time.

When you add resistance training to your lower body workouts, such as lifting weights or using resistance bands, you stimulate muscle growth, also known as hypertrophy. Stronger and more developed leg muscles mean that your body will burn more calories even when you're not working out. This metabolic boost aids in creating a "fat-burning effect" that works in the background, helping you burn more calories throughout the day.

- **Metabolism-Boosting Exercises**: Focus on resistance exercises like deadlifts, leg presses, and weighted step-ups to stimulate leg muscle growth and increase your resting metabolic rate.

3. The Power of Excess Post-Exercise Oxygen Consumption (EPOC)

The concept of excess post-exercise oxygen consumption, or EPOC, is also known as the "afterburn effect." After an intense lower body workout, your body needs extra oxygen to restore itself to a resting state, repair muscles, and replenish energy stores. This process requires additional energy, meaning you continue to burn calories for hours after your workout has ended.

Lower body exercises that involve high intensity or a high volume of reps—especially those that engage multiple muscle groups—are particularly effective at increasing EPOC. Workouts that include movements like jump squats, plyometric lunges, or high-intensity interval training (HIIT) circuits can amplify EPOC, enhancing the total caloric burn and contributing to faster fat loss.

- **EPOC-Enhancing Workouts**: Incorporate plyometric exercises like box jumps, jump lunges, and HIIT circuits involving lower body exercises to maximize the afterburn effect.

4. Targeted Fat Burning and Body Composition Changes

While it's a common misconception that you can "spot reduce" fat from specific areas, lower body workouts do help tone and sculpt the legs, hips, and glutes, which contributes to an overall leaner appearance. As you build lean muscle mass, your body composition improves, leading to a lower body fat percentage over time.

Lower body training also plays a role in hormonal responses that promote fat loss. Research shows that heavy, compound exercises stimulate the release of growth hormone and testosterone, both of which are critical for fat metabolism and muscle building. These hormones help your body tap into stored fat as an energy source and promote muscle preservation, which is particularly helpful during a calorie deficit for weight loss.

- **Exercises for Body Composition**: Strength exercises like Bulgarian split squats, single-leg deadlifts, and weighted lunges are great for building muscle and creating a leaner lower body shape.

5. Sustained Fat Loss and Weight Maintenance

Leg workouts not only help with immediate calorie burn but also contribute to sustainable fat loss and weight maintenance. Building a routine that consistently targets the lower body can improve metabolic flexibility, allowing your body to better utilize stored fat as fuel. Consistent lower body training creates long-term adaptations in your metabolism, which supports sustainable weight management.

Additionally, leg workouts tend to be highly motivating and empowering, often making it easier to stick to a regular exercise routine. This is a crucial factor for sustained weight loss, as adherence to a consistent workout program is one of the most important predictors of long-term success in managing body weight and maintaining a lean physique.

- **Exercises for Long-Term Fat Loss**: Movements like squats, deadlifts, and lunges that can be progressively loaded and varied over time are excellent for building a sustainable, effective workout routine.

Lower body workouts are a powerful component of a comprehensive weight loss and fat-burning plan. By engaging large muscle groups in the hips, thighs, and glutes, you create a high calorie burn, boost your metabolism, and take advantage of the afterburn effect (EPOC). Consistently training the lower body not only helps reduce body fat but also supports long-term weight maintenance and a leaner body composition. Through effective lower body training, you can achieve a strong, toned physique while enhancing your metabolic health and creating a foundation for lasting fitness success.

Chapter 3: Getting Started – Goal Setting and Motivation

This chapter provides a roadmap for readers to set meaningful fitness goals, maintain motivation, and track their progress effectively. Goal setting is one of the most important aspects of a successful workout program, and knowing how to set realistic and achievable targets makes all the difference. By understanding how to define personal fitness goals, readers can make the journey enjoyable, measurable, and rewarding.

---

1. Define Your Goals: Tips for Setting Realistic Fitness Goals

Setting clear, realistic goals is the first step toward transforming your lower body and overall fitness. Understanding your personal motivations and objectives can guide you in selecting the right type of training and tracking your progress.

Types of Fitness Goals:

- **Strength**: Many people seek to improve their lower body strength, which is crucial for overall functionality, mobility, and injury prevention. Stronger legs also support heavier lifts, reduce strain on joints, and improve stability.
- **Tone**: For those aiming for a lean, sculpted appearance, focusing on toning exercises

can help. Toning goals often emphasize higher-repetition exercises with moderate weights or body weight, which encourages muscle definition without adding excessive bulk.

- **Endurance**: Building endurance is essential for those who want stamina for long-lasting workouts or sports that demand continuous lower body activity, like running or cycling. Endurance goals emphasize cardiovascular health, muscular stamina, and mental resilience.
- **Combination**: Some people aim to combine multiple goals—such as building strength while enhancing muscle tone or balancing endurance with power. This approach requires a well-rounded workout plan with a variety of exercises and training techniques.

Setting SMART Goals: To make goals actionable, it's helpful to follow the SMART method:

- **Specific**: Define your goal in clear, precise terms. (e.g., "Increase my squat weight by 10 lbs within three months.")
- **Measurable**: Choose goals that you can track and measure, whether it's reps, weights, or inches lost.
- **Achievable**: Set goals that are challenging but within reach to maintain motivation and avoid burnout.

- **Relevant**: Ensure your goals align with your broader fitness vision and lifestyle.
- **Time-Bound**: Attach a timeline to your goals, such as 4 weeks, 3 months, or a year, to help you stay accountable and track progress effectively.

Tips for Defining Goals:

- Start small if you're new to lower body workouts, setting short-term goals (e.g., mastering proper squat form) before expanding to more challenging targets.
- Write down your goals to keep yourself accountable.
- Adjust your goals over time based on your progress and changing interests or needs.

---

2. Tracking Your Progress: Measuring Results for Motivation and Consistency

Tracking progress is one of the most effective ways to stay motivated and focused. By measuring results consistently, you can see tangible evidence of your hard work and make necessary adjustments along the way. Tracking also helps to build momentum and keep you committed.

Methods for Tracking Progress:

- **Photos**: Progress photos offer a visual record of your transformation over time.

Consider taking photos from different angles (front, side, and back) every 4-6 weeks to notice changes in muscle tone, size, and symmetry.

- **Measurements**: Using a tape measure to track the circumference of your hips, thighs, calves, and waist can provide a quantitative view of your progress. Muscle gain, fat loss, or a combination will show up in these measurements.
- **Strength Tests**: Periodic strength testing can help you assess improvements in your lifts, endurance, and stability. Record your baseline performance for key exercises like squats, lunges, and deadlifts, and test your limits every 4-6 weeks to evaluate your progress.
- **Workout Logs**: Keep a workout journal or use a fitness app to log details about each workout, such as sets, reps, weights, and exercise variations. Over time, this data will help you see trends, identify areas for improvement, and notice gains in strength and endurance.

Tips for Consistent Tracking:

- **Set Regular Checkpoints**: Schedule regular check-ins, whether weekly or monthly, to review your goals and track your progress.
- **Use Technology**: Many fitness apps provide progress-tracking features and can

store data on your workouts, measurements, and photos.

- **Celebrate Small Wins**: Acknowledging small victories, such as a new personal record in deadlifts or visible muscle definition, can boost motivation and confidence.
- **Adapt as Needed**: If your progress plateaus or your goals shift, adjust your workouts or tracking methods to align with your evolving fitness journey.

By the end of this chapter, readers will have a clear understanding of how to set specific, realistic goals tailored to their unique fitness aspirations and how to track their progress in a meaningful way. With clear goals and consistent tracking, every workout becomes a step toward a stronger, more toned lower body—and a boost in confidence. The journey begins with a solid foundation in goal-setting and motivation, ensuring long-term success and making the path to "legs for days" achievable and enjoyable.

Building a Positive Mindset: Motivation Techniques to Keep Going Even When Progress Feels Slow

Building a positive mindset is essential for sticking with a fitness routine and achieving long-term success. During any fitness journey, there will be times when progress feels slow or even nonexistent. Knowing how to cultivate a resilient and positive mindset can keep you moving forward, even during challenging periods. In this section, we'll explore strategies and techniques to help you stay motivated, celebrate small wins, and embrace the journey toward a stronger, toned lower body.

---

1. Focus on the Journey, Not Just the Destination

One of the best ways to stay motivated is to shift your perspective from only focusing on the end result to appreciating the process. Embracing the journey helps you find joy in daily actions and the small steps that lead to transformation over time. Instead of being discouraged by slow progress, see each workout as an opportunity to challenge yourself, learn, and grow.

- **Technique**: Reflect on your personal reasons for starting this journey. Write down why having strong, toned legs is meaningful to you. Maybe it's about feeling more confident, improving your health, or building resilience. Revisit these reasons when you need a reminder of your motivation.

---

2. Set Micro-Goals and Celebrate Small Wins

While having big goals is essential, breaking them down into smaller, more achievable "micro-goals" can help sustain motivation. Each small victory builds momentum, giving you a series of achievements to look forward to instead of waiting for a single, final outcome. These micro-goals might include increasing your squat weight by five pounds, completing a workout without pausing, or hitting a new personal best on a challenging exercise.

- **Technique**: At the start of each week, set one or two small goals specific to your workouts. This could be anything from improving your form on a new exercise to adding an extra set of reps. At the end of the week, celebrate these wins, whether it's treating yourself to something special or simply acknowledging your progress with pride.

3. Practice Positive Self-Talk and Visualization

Your inner dialogue has a significant impact on motivation and performance. When progress feels slow, it's easy to fall into a cycle of negative self-talk, which can lead to self-doubt or giving up. Practicing positive self-talk and visualization helps you combat these doubts by reinforcing self-belief, resilience, and determination. Visualization can be particularly powerful, as it involves mentally rehearsing success and seeing yourself achieve your goals.

- **Technique**: Before each workout, take a few moments to visualize yourself successfully completing the exercises. Picture yourself stronger, with toned legs, and feel the sense of accomplishment. During workouts, if you start to feel discouraged, replace negative thoughts ("I can't do this") with positive affirmations ("I'm getting stronger with each rep").

4. Track Non-Scale Victories (NSVs)

While physical changes like muscle tone and strength are measurable, there are many non-physical benefits that come from consistent exercise. These are called non-scale victories (NSVs), and they can be highly motivating. NSVs can include improved mood, increased energy, better sleep, or the ability to perform daily tasks more easily. Recognizing these benefits helps remind you that progress isn't only about the visible outcomes.

- **Technique**: Keep a journal to record your NSVs. Each week, write down at least one positive change you've noticed, even if it's something as simple as feeling more energetic. Revisiting these entries can boost motivation, especially during periods when visual progress is less apparent.

5. Surround Yourself with Positive Influence

The people around you can significantly influence your motivation and mindset. Surrounding yourself with supportive individuals who understand and encourage your goals can help keep you inspired, accountable, and focused. Whether it's friends, family, a workout partner, or an online fitness community, connecting with others on a similar journey can provide motivation, share insights, and offer a sense of camaraderie.

- **Technique**: If possible, find a workout partner or join a fitness group, either in-person or online. Share your goals, celebrate each other's victories, and lean on each other when motivation dips. Positive influence from others can reinforce your dedication and give you a boost on days when you need it.

6. Learn to Appreciate Rest and Recovery

Rest days are an essential part of any fitness journey, as they allow your muscles to recover and grow stronger. When you feel impatient for results, it's easy to push yourself too hard, which can lead to burnout, fatigue, or injury. By embracing rest and recovery, you honor your body's needs and create a sustainable approach to reaching your goals.

- **Technique**: Schedule rest days and treat them as part of the process, not time off from it. On these days, practice light activities like stretching or yoga, or simply take time to relax. Remind yourself that rest days are essential to your success, allowing you to return to your workouts stronger and more energized.

---

7. Accept Plateaus and Use Them as Learning Moments

Plateaus are a natural part of any fitness journey. While they can be frustrating, they're also an opportunity to re-evaluate your approach, adjust your routine, or incorporate new challenges. A plateau doesn't mean failure; it's a chance to fine-tune your training and reflect on how far you've already come.

- **Technique**: When progress slows, don't give up—instead, assess your routine and consider small changes to stimulate growth, such as increasing weights, altering reps, or trying new exercises. Use this time to celebrate the strength you've already built and trust that with persistence, you'll break through.

Building a positive mindset is the foundation of a successful fitness journey. By focusing on the process, setting small goals, practicing positive self-talk, and celebrating non-scale victories, you'll find that motivation becomes easier to sustain, even when progress feels slow. Embrace each step of the journey and remember that every effort, no matter how small, brings you closer to achieving strong, toned legs—and the confidence and satisfaction that come with it.

Part 2: Power-Packed Lower Body Exercises

Chapter 4: Essential Hip and Thigh Exercises

This chapter focuses on foundational exercises that target the hips and thighs using only your body weight. These exercises are highly effective for building strength, stability, and endurance in the lower body and are accessible to everyone, regardless of fitness level. Bodyweight exercises allow you to master form, build strength, and gain confidence before progressing to weighted movements. Let's dive into some essential exercises that lay the groundwork for a toned, powerful lower body.

Bodyweight Basics: Foundational Moves for Lower Body Strength

1. Squats

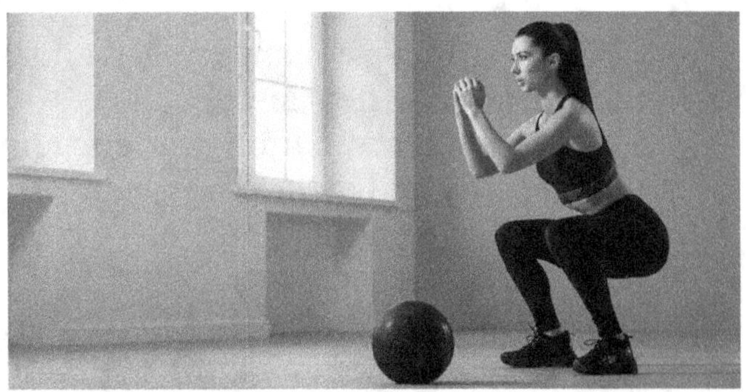

- **Overview**: Squats are one of the best all-around exercises for developing the quadriceps, glutes, hamstrings, and core. This simple yet powerful movement engages multiple muscle groups, improves balance, and builds strength.
- **How to Perform**:
  1. Stand with feet shoulder-width apart, toes pointed slightly outward.
  2. Lower your hips down and back as if sitting in a chair, keeping your chest up and knees in line with your toes.
  3. Lower until your thighs are parallel to the ground or as far as comfortable.
  4. Drive through your heels to stand back up.
- **Benefits**: Builds strength, improves mobility, and serves as a foundation for weighted squats.

2. **Lunges**
- **Overview**: Lunges work the quadriceps, hamstrings, glutes, and calves. They also challenge stability and coordination by engaging the core and balance muscles.
- **How to Perform**:
  1. Stand upright and take a step forward with one leg, lowering your hips until both knees are bent at a 90-degree angle.

2. Your front knee should be directly above your ankle, and your back knee should hover just above the ground.
3. Push through the heel of your front foot to return to the starting position.

- **Variations**: Walking lunges, reverse lunges, and side lunges to target different parts of the lower body.
- **Benefits**: Increases strength and stability, improves balance, and is easily modified to add challenge.

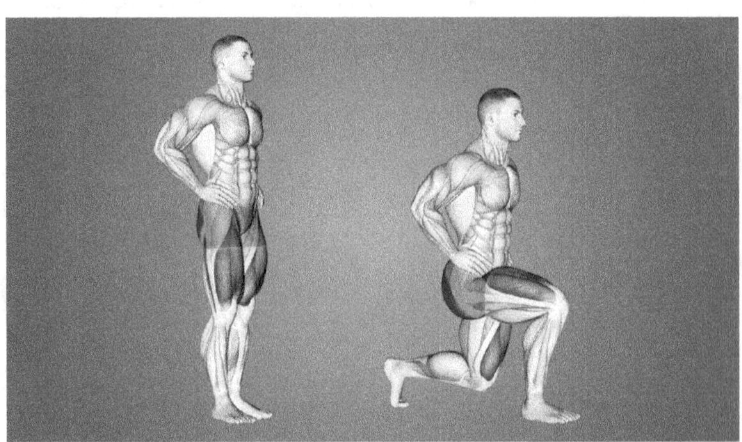

3. **Glute Bridges**
   - **Overview**: Glute bridges primarily target the glutes and hamstrings while also engaging the core. This movement is excellent for isolating the glutes, especially for those looking to strengthen and shape the backside.

- o **How to Perform**:
    1. Lie on your back with knees bent and feet flat on the ground, hip-width apart.
    2. Tighten your core, squeeze your glutes, and lift your hips toward the ceiling until your body forms a straight line from your knees to your shoulders.
    3. Lower your hips back down to the ground with control.
  - o **Benefits**: Strengthens glutes and hamstrings, improves pelvic stability, and can relieve lower back tension.

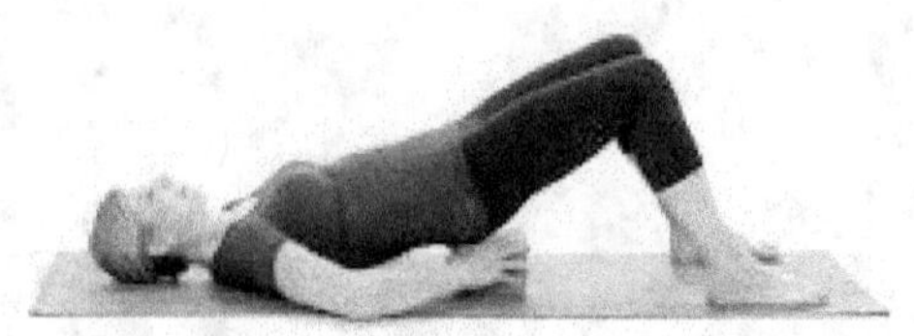

4. **Side-Lying Leg Lifts**
   - o **Overview**: This exercise isolates the hip abductors, which help with stability, balance, and lateral movements.
   - o **How to Perform**:

1. Lie on your side with legs stacked and straighten your bottom arm to support your head.
2. Raise your top leg toward the ceiling, keeping your hips stable and toes pointing forward.
3. Lower your leg back down with control and repeat.

- **Benefits**: Tones the outer thighs and hips, improves hip stability, and builds endurance in smaller stabilizing muscles.

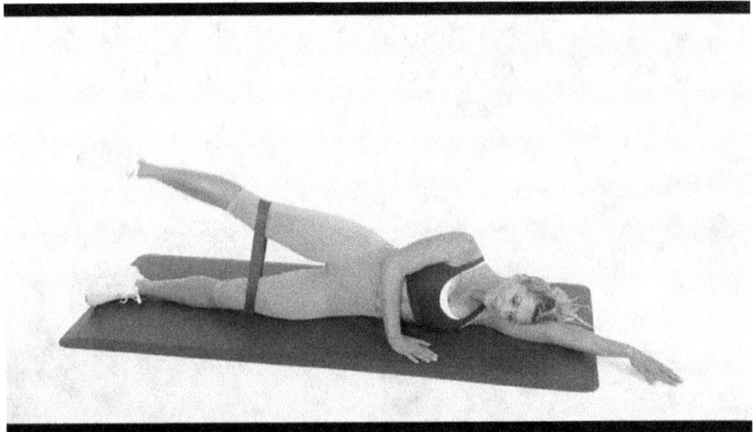

5. Bulgarian Split Squats

- **Overview**: The Bulgarian split squat is a unilateral exercise that targets the quadriceps, glutes, and hamstrings. This advanced variation of the lunge challenges balance and

stability while emphasizing the front leg's muscles.
- **How to Perform**:
  1. Stand a few feet in front of a bench or step and place the top of one foot behind you on the bench.
  2. Lower your back knee toward the ground while keeping your front knee aligned over your ankle.
  3. Push through the heel of your front foot to return to the starting position.
- **Benefits**: Builds lower body strength, improves balance, and corrects muscle imbalances between legs.

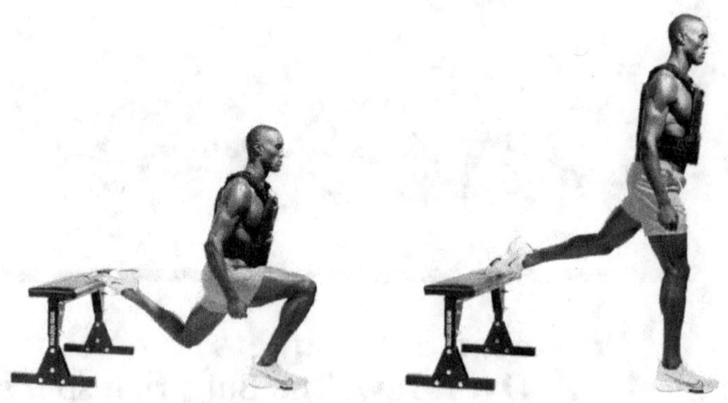

6. **Step-Ups**
   - **Overview**: Step-ups strengthen the quadriceps, glutes, and hamstrings while enhancing balance and

stability. They mimic real-life movements, making them practical for daily activities.

- o **How to Perform**:
    1. Stand in front of a sturdy bench or platform.
    2. Step up with one leg, pressing through your heel to lift your body onto the platform.
    3. Step back down with control and repeat on the opposite leg.
- o **Benefits**: Improves strength, balance, and stability in the lower body, and helps increase unilateral strength.

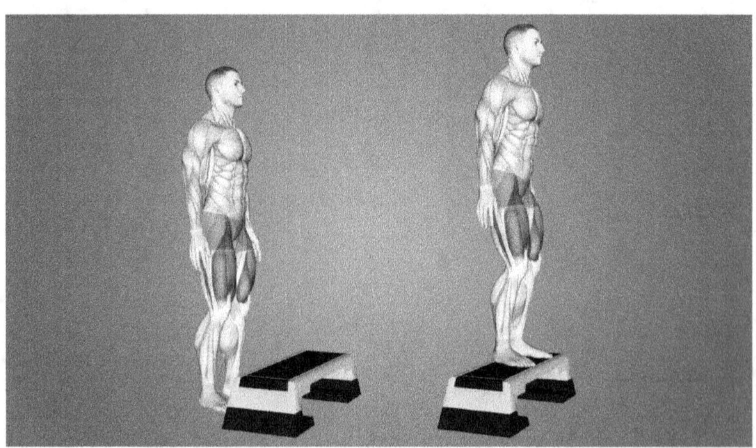

7. **Calf Raises**
    - o **Overview**: Calf raises isolate the calf muscles and are important for balance and stability. They're especially useful for those looking to strengthen the lower legs.

o **How to Perform**:
  1. Stand with feet hip-width apart, and slowly lift your heels, balancing on the balls of your feet.
  2. Pause at the top, then slowly lower your heels back down.
o **Benefits**: Builds calf strength, improves balance, and enhances muscle endurance in the lower legs.

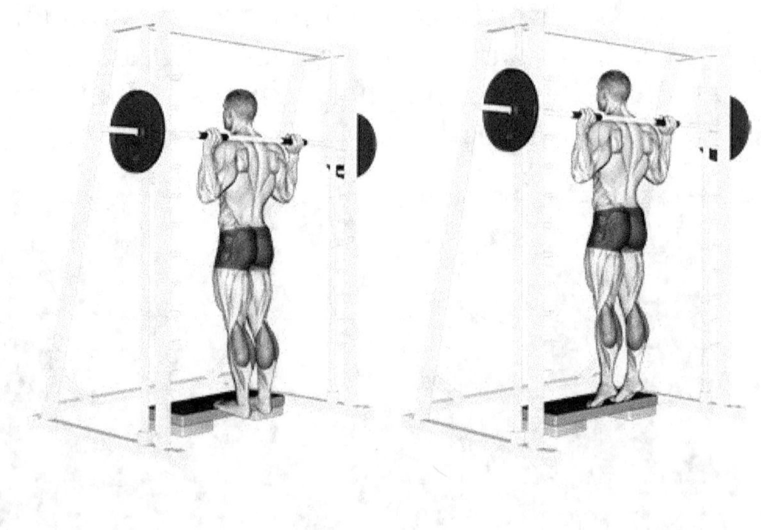

Tips for Maximizing Bodyweight Exercises

- **Focus on Form**: Proper form ensures that you're targeting the intended muscles and helps prevent injury.
- **Control Your Movements**: Slow, controlled movements activate muscles

more effectively than rushing through repetitions.

- **Add Variations for Challenge**: Once comfortable with these basics, try different variations like tempo changes, single-leg versions, or adding elevation.
- **Mind-Muscle Connection**: Concentrate on the muscles being worked to enhance engagement and maximize effectiveness.

These foundational exercises lay the groundwork for building strength and stability in the hips, thighs, and glutes. Mastering these movements will set you up for success as you progress into more advanced lower body routines throughout the book. Whether you're just starting out or refining your technique, these bodyweight basics provide the essential building blocks for a powerful, sculpted lower body.

Dumbbell and Kettlebell Variations: Adding Resistance for Strength, Growth, and Power

Incorporating dumbbells and kettlebells into your hip and thigh workouts is a fantastic way to build muscle, increase power, and enhance overall strength. The added resistance intensifies the workout, challenging your muscles to work harder, which leads to growth and improved endurance. Here's a look at key exercises that target the lower body using these versatile weights, with guidance on form and benefits.

1. Goblet Squats

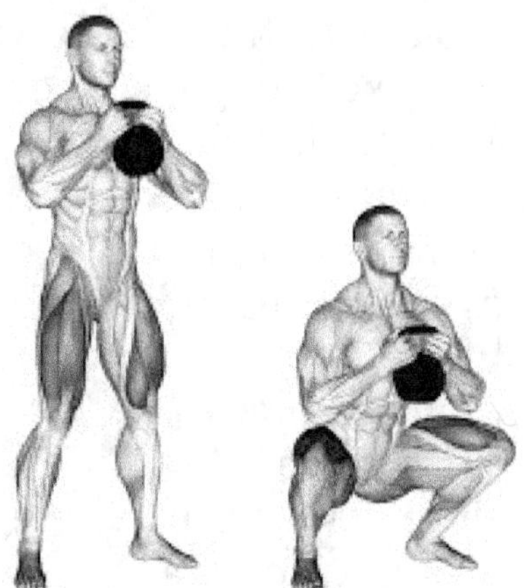

- **Overview**: The goblet squat is a variation of the traditional squat where you hold a dumbbell or kettlebell close to your chest. This position activates the core while targeting the quadriceps, glutes, and hamstrings.
- **How to Perform**:
    1. Hold a dumbbell or kettlebell vertically at chest level with both hands, keeping elbows close to your body.
    2. Stand with feet shoulder-width apart, toes slightly pointed outward.
    3. Lower into a squat, pushing your hips back and bending your knees until your thighs are parallel to the ground.

4. Press through your heels to return to the starting position.

- **Benefits**: Builds lower body strength, promotes core engagement, and enhances mobility through the hips.

2. Dumbbell Deadlifts

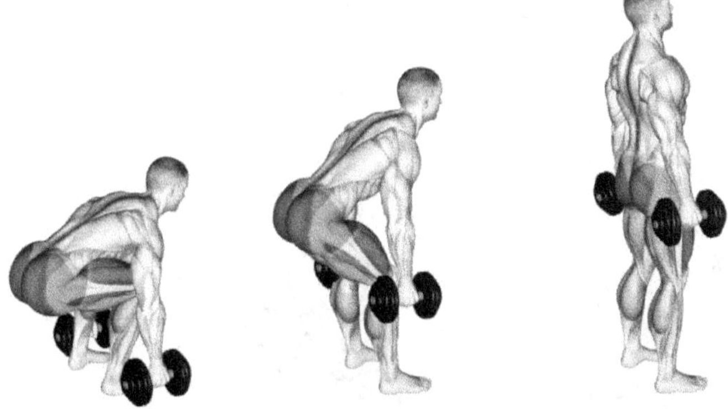

- **Overview**: Dumbbell deadlifts target the hamstrings, glutes, and lower back. This exercise is excellent for building posterior chain strength and improving hip mobility.
- **How to Perform**:
  1. Stand with feet hip-width apart, holding a dumbbell in each hand in front of your thighs, palms facing you.
  2. Keeping a slight bend in your knees, hinge at the hips and lower the dumbbells toward the ground, keeping your back flat.

3. Squeeze your glutes and hamstrings to return to the starting position, bringing the weights back to hip level.

- **Benefits**: Strengthens the glutes, hamstrings, and core while enhancing flexibility in the hips and lower back.

3. Bulgarian Split Squats

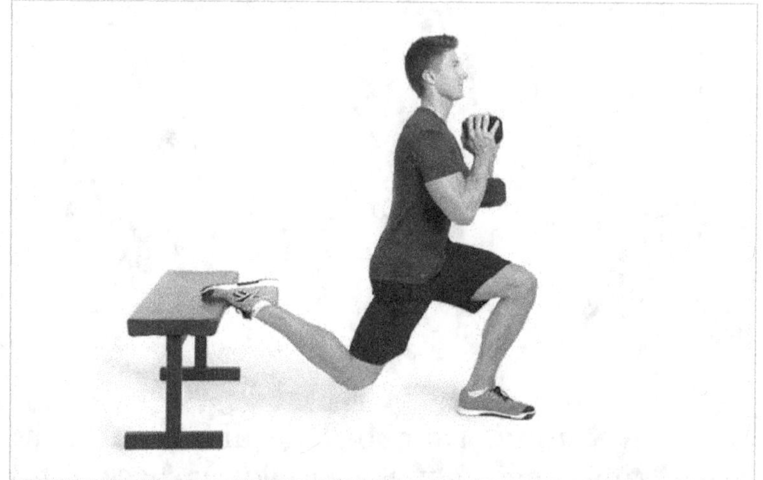

- **Overview**: Adding a dumbbell or kettlebell to Bulgarian split squats intensifies the exercise, helping to build unilateral (one-sided) strength and balance. This move targets the glutes, quads, and hamstrings with a strong emphasis on balance.
- **How to Perform**:
    1. Stand a few feet in front of a bench or platform, holding a dumbbell in each hand.

2. Place one foot behind you on the bench, laces down, and position the other foot forward.
3. Lower your back knee toward the floor until your front thigh is parallel to the ground, keeping your chest up and back straight.
4. Push through the heel of your front foot to return to the starting position.

- **Benefits**: Improves leg strength, balance, and stability, and helps correct muscular imbalances between legs.

4. Kettlebell Swings

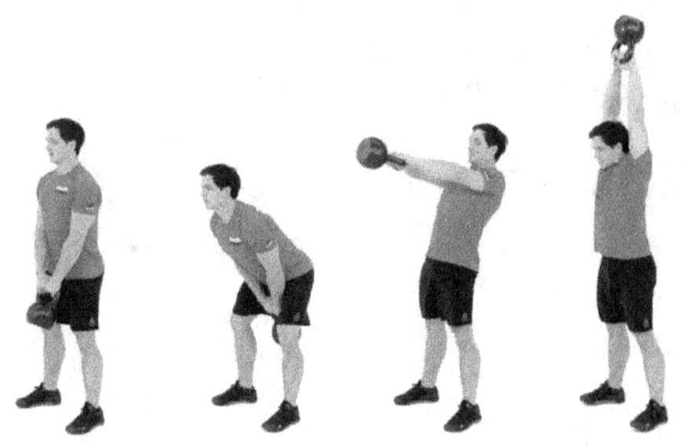

- **Overview**: The kettlebell swing is a dynamic, full-body movement that builds explosive power in the hips, glutes, and hamstrings. It also improves cardiovascular endurance and works the core.
- **How to Perform**:

1. Stand with feet shoulder-width apart, holding a kettlebell with both hands in front of your hips.
2. Bend slightly at the knees and hinge at the hips, swinging the kettlebell back between your legs.
3. Drive through your hips to swing the kettlebell up to shoulder height, using momentum rather than arm strength.
4. Control the descent of the kettlebell, allowing it to swing back between your legs, then repeat.

- **Benefits**: Builds explosive power, enhances hip mobility, and improves cardiovascular fitness while targeting the glutes and hamstrings.

5. Dumbbell Step-Ups

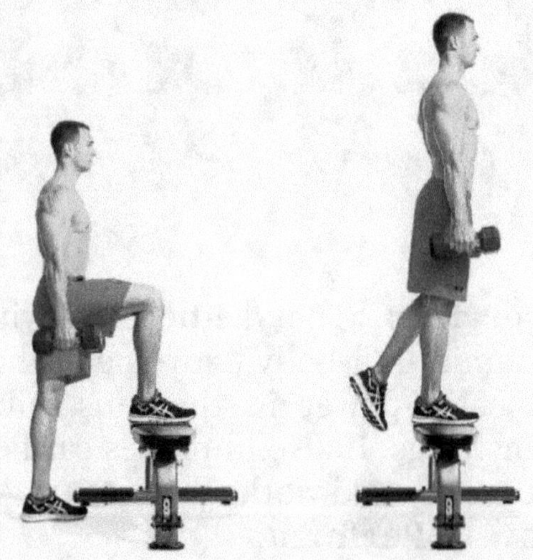

- **Overview**: Step-ups with dumbbells add an extra challenge to the bodyweight step-up, focusing on the glutes, quads, and hamstrings while improving balance and coordination.
- **How to Perform**:
  1. Stand in front of a platform or bench, holding a dumbbell in each hand at your sides.
  2. Step onto the platform with one foot, pressing through the heel to lift your body up.
  3. Step back down with control and repeat on the opposite leg.
- **Benefits**: Strengthens the legs and glutes, improves stability, and mimics real-life movements like climbing stairs.

7. Kettlebell Goblet Lunges

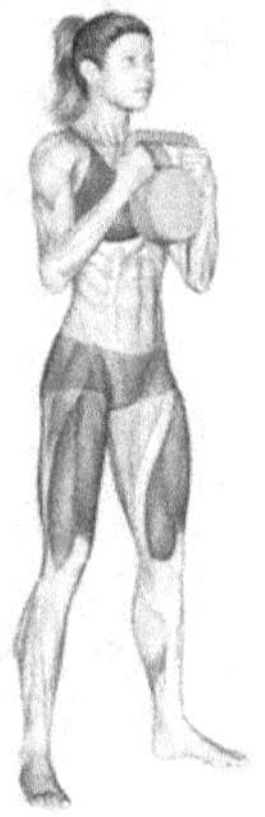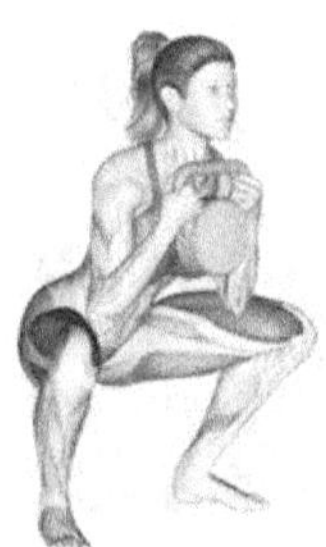

- **Overview**: This exercise combines the core stability of the goblet hold with the lower body challenge of lunges, targeting the quads, glutes, and hamstrings.

- **How to Perform**:
    1. Hold a kettlebell at chest level with both hands, similar to the goblet squat.
    2. Step forward with one foot, lowering into a lunge until both knees are bent at 90-degree angles.
    3. Push off the front foot to return to the starting position and repeat with the opposite leg.
- **Benefits**: Builds lower body strength and endurance, improves core stability, and enhances balance.

7. Dumbbell Sumo Squats

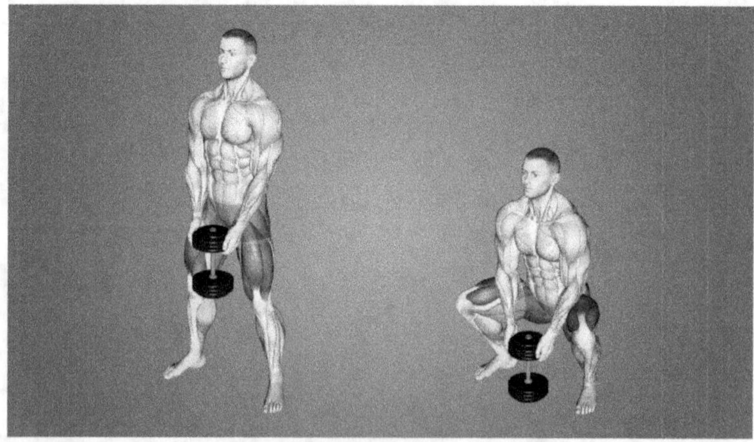

- **Overview**: The sumo squat variation with a dumbbell targets the inner thighs and glutes more than the standard squat, thanks to the wider stance.

- **How to Perform**:
    1. Stand with feet wider than shoulder-width apart, toes pointing out, and hold a dumbbell in both hands.
    2. Lower into a squat, keeping your back straight and core tight.
    3. Push through your heels to stand back up, squeezing your glutes at the top.
- **Benefits**: Strengthens the inner thighs and glutes, improves hip mobility, and increases stability in the lower body.

Tips for Maximizing Dumbbell and Kettlebell Workouts

- **Start Light and Progress Gradually**: Begin with a manageable weight to ensure proper form, then increase gradually to build strength.
- **Focus on Form**: Keeping your form strict is crucial to prevent injury and ensure you're targeting the right muscles.
- **Incorporate Variations**: Experiment with different exercises and weights to keep workouts challenging and engaging.
- **Listen to Your Body**: Ensure you're not overloading and take rest days to allow for muscle recovery.

Adding dumbbells and kettlebells to your lower body routine takes your strength and muscle growth to the next level. These exercises improve both power and endurance while helping you achieve a toned, sculpted look. With these variations in your arsenal, you'll have everything you need to transform your lower body with power, shape, and strength.

Machine-Based Exercises: Targeted Strength and Isolation

Machine-based exercises offer a controlled, effective way to target specific muscles in the hips and thighs. These exercises are ideal for isolating individual muscle groups, allowing you to focus on areas that might need extra attention or strength. Using gym machines can also provide stability, making it easier to focus on muscle engagement without the balance challenges that free weights might present. Here's a look at key machine exercises to add to your lower body routine.

1. Leg Press

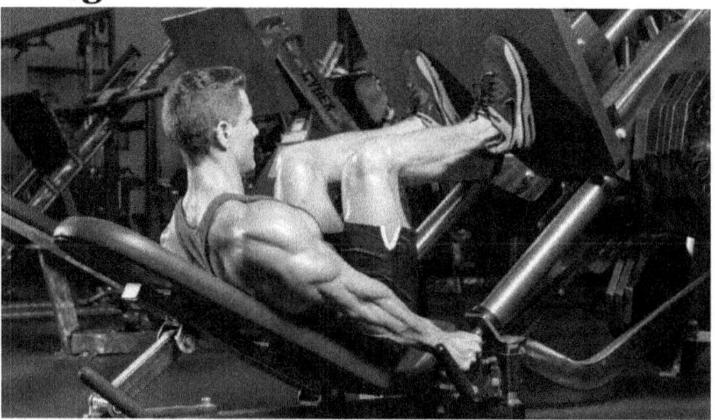

- **Overview**: The leg press machine is a staple for building lower body strength, particularly in the quadriceps, glutes, and hamstrings. The seated position allows you to press significant weight while minimizing strain on your back.
- **How to Perform**:
    1. Sit on the leg press machine and position your feet shoulder-width apart on the platform.
    2. Engage your core, release the safety handles, and press the weight up to straighten your legs without locking your knees.
    3. Slowly lower the weight by bending your knees toward your chest until they form a 90-degree angle.
    4. Press through your heels to return to the starting position.
- **Benefits**: Strengthens the entire lower body, increases quad and glute power, and allows for progressive weight increases.

2. Leg Extension

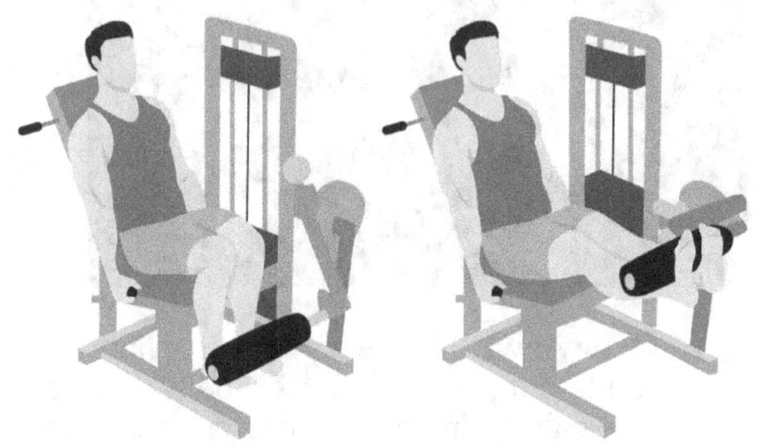

- **Overview**: The leg extension machine is designed to isolate the quadriceps, helping to define and strengthen the front of the thighs. This exercise is highly effective for building knee joint stability and muscular endurance in the quads.
- **How to Perform**:
    1. Sit on the leg extension machine, adjusting the pad so it rests on the front of your ankles.
    2. Grip the handles and straighten your legs, lifting the weight by contracting your quadriceps.

3. Pause briefly at the top, then lower the weight back to the starting position with control.
- **Benefits**: Isolates the quadriceps for targeted strength and endurance, improves knee stability, and enhances muscle definition in the front thighs.

3. Seated Leg Curl

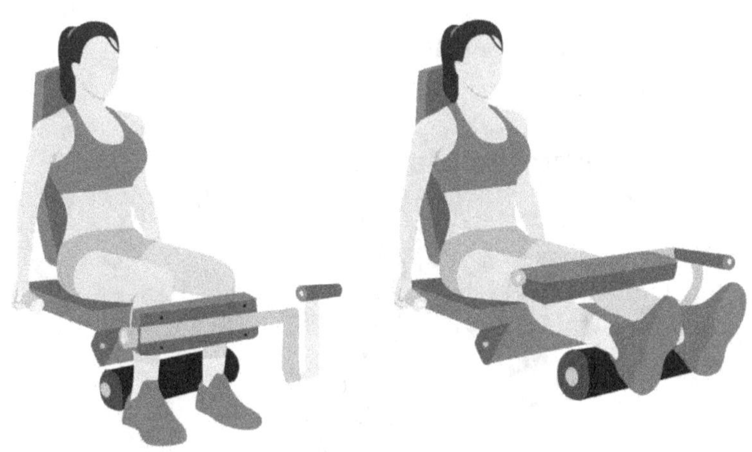

- **Overview**: The seated leg curl machine targets the hamstrings, strengthening the muscles along the back of your thighs. This exercise is great for developing hamstring endurance and flexibility.
- **How to Perform**:

1. Sit on the machine, positioning the pad above your ankles with your back against the seat.
2. Grasp the handles and pull the pad down by bending your knees, engaging your hamstrings to lift the weight.
3. Lower the weight back up slowly, keeping control throughout the movement.

- **Benefits**: Builds hamstring strength, enhances balance with quad-dominant exercises, and improves lower body stability.

4. Hip Abductor Machine

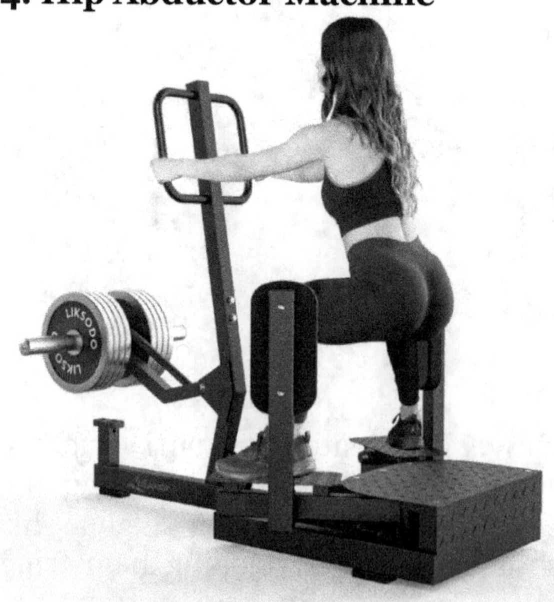

- **Overview**: The hip abductor machine targets the muscles on the outer hips and thighs, particularly the gluteus medius and minimus. This exercise helps with balance and stability in movements like squats and lunges.

- **How to Perform**:
    1. Sit on the hip abductor machine, placing your knees against the outer pads.
    2. Grip the handles and press outward with your legs, squeezing the glutes and outer thighs.
    3. Pause briefly at the top, then slowly bring your legs back to the starting position.
- **Benefits**: Strengthens the outer thighs and hips, improves balance, and adds definition to the glutes.

5. Glute Kickback Machine

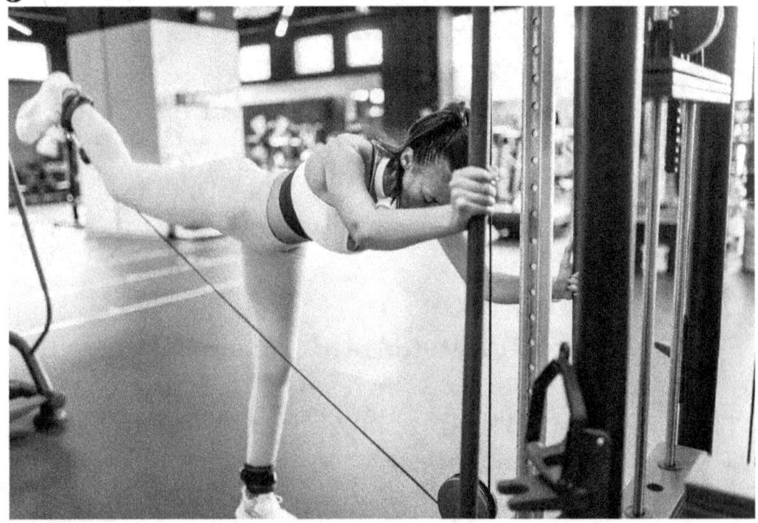

- **Overview**: The glute kickback machine is a targeted exercise that emphasizes the gluteus maximus, helping to sculpt and strengthen the glutes and improve hip extension strength.
- **How to Perform**:
  1. Position yourself on the machine, bracing your chest against the pad and placing one foot on the platform.
  2. Engage your core and push the platform back by extending your leg, squeezing your glute at the top of the movement.
  3. Lower back down with control, then switch legs.
- **Benefits**: Isolates the glutes, enhances hip strength, and helps create a rounder, more defined glute shape.

6. Smith Machine Squats

- **Overview**: The Smith machine provides a stabilized bar path for squats, making it easier to focus on the quadriceps, glutes, and hamstrings without worrying about balance.
- **How to Perform**:
  1. Stand under the bar on the Smith machine with feet shoulder-width apart and bar resting across your shoulders.
  2. Lower into a squat, keeping your back straight and chest up.

3. Push through your heels to return to the starting position.
  - **Benefits**: Builds lower body strength in a controlled, safe way; great for beginners or those recovering from injury.

Tips for Maximizing Machine-Based Exercises

- **Adjust Machine Settings**: Ensure each machine is set up to fit your body dimensions, allowing for full range of motion.
- **Start with a Warm-Up**: Warm up with a few minutes of cardio and dynamic stretching to prepare your muscles.
- **Focus on Muscle Engagement**: Since machines reduce balance requirements, focus on isolating and engaging the target muscles.
- **Progress Gradually**: Increase the weight incrementally to build strength without risking injury.

Machine-based exercises provide stability and control, making them excellent for isolating muscles and ensuring consistent form. They're a valuable addition to any lower body routine and can be used to build foundational strength before moving to more complex, free-weight exercises.

Chapter 5: Glute-Focused Moves for Lift and Shape

Achieving a well-rounded lower body workout requires focused attention on the glutes, the powerhouse muscles that support hip stability, posture, and athletic performance. This chapter explores a selection of highly effective glute exercises designed to target and engage these muscles, enhancing shape, lift, and strength. Incorporating these glute-focused exercises into your routine will not only improve the look of your lower body but also contribute to greater lower body stability and injury prevention.

Effective Glute Exercises

1. **Hip Thrusts**

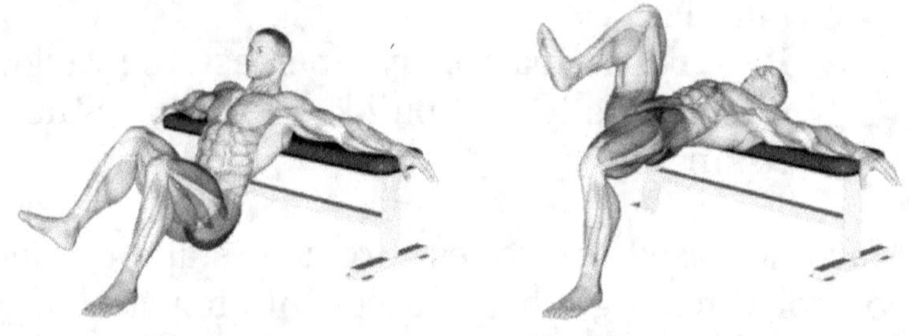

- **Overview**: Hip thrusts are one of the best exercises for isolating and strengthening the glutes. By allowing a full range of motion and direct focus on the glutes, hip thrusts enhance shape and lift.

- **How to Perform**:
    1. Sit on the floor with your upper back resting against a bench and feet flat on the ground.
    2. Place a barbell or weighted plate across your hips for added resistance.
    3. Drive through your heels, lifting your hips toward the ceiling and squeezing your glutes at the top.
    4. Lower your hips back down with control and repeat.
- **Benefits**: Directly targets the glutes, increases glute strength and size, and helps improve hip stability and power.

2. **Glute Bridges**

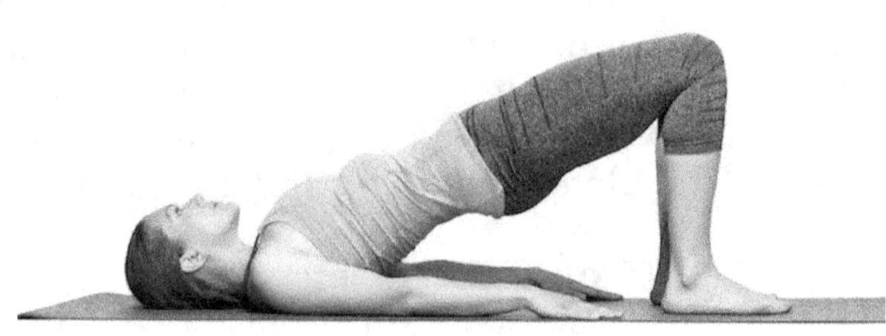

o **Overview**: Glute bridges are similar to hip thrusts but performed from a lying position on the floor. This exercise activates the glutes and hamstrings, making it ideal for building foundational glute strength.

o **How to Perform**:
1. Lie on your back with knees bent and feet flat on the floor, hip-width apart.
2. Engage your core and lift your hips by pressing through your heels, squeezing your glutes at the top.
3. Lower back down slowly, maintaining control.

o **Benefits**: Strengthens the glutes and hamstrings, improves hip flexibility, and provides a good warm-up for heavier glute exercises.

3. **Step-Ups**

o **Overview**: Step-ups are a unilateral (one-legged) exercise that works the glutes, hamstrings, and quads while also improving balance and coordination. By stepping onto an elevated surface, you engage the glutes in a natural, functional movement.

o **How to Perform**:
1. Stand in front of a sturdy bench or box.
2. Place one foot on the platform, pressing through your heel to

lift your body onto the bench, bringing your other foot up to meet it.

3. Step back down with control and switch legs.

- **Benefits**: Builds glute strength, improves balance and coordination, and enhances lower body functionality for daily movements.

4. **Bulgarian Split Squats**

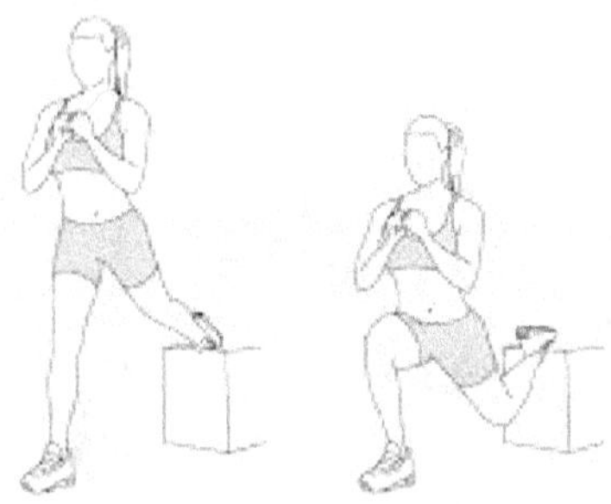

- **Overview**: The Bulgarian split squat is a powerful lower body exercise that activates the glutes, quadriceps, and hamstrings. Elevating one foot targets the glutes more effectively and adds an element of balance.
- **How to Perform**:
    1. Stand a few feet in front of a bench, placing one foot behind you on the bench.

2. Lower your body into a squat
   position, keeping your torso
   upright.
3. Press through the heel of your
   front foot to return to
   standing, engaging the glute on
   your working leg.
- o **Benefits**: Intensely targets the
  glutes and thighs, improves balance,
  and enhances unilateral strength.

5. **Romanian Deadlifts**

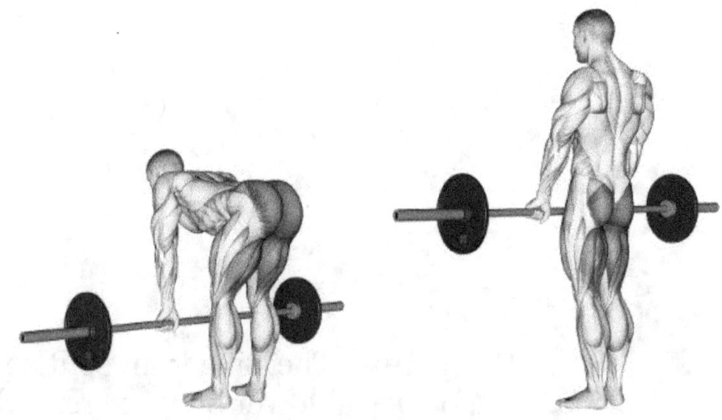

- o **Overview**: Romanian deadlifts
  (RDLs) emphasize the hamstrings
  and glutes, building strength in the
  posterior chain (the muscles along
  the backside of your body) and
  improving hip mobility.
- o **How to Perform**:

1. Stand with feet hip-width apart, holding dumbbells or a barbell in front of your thighs.
2. Keeping a slight bend in your knees, hinge at the hips to lower the weight, maintaining a straight back.
3. Stop when you feel a stretch in your hamstrings, then return to standing by engaging your glutes.

- **Benefits**: Strengthens the glutes and hamstrings, promotes hip mobility, and builds posterior chain strength.

6. **Cable Pull-Throughs**

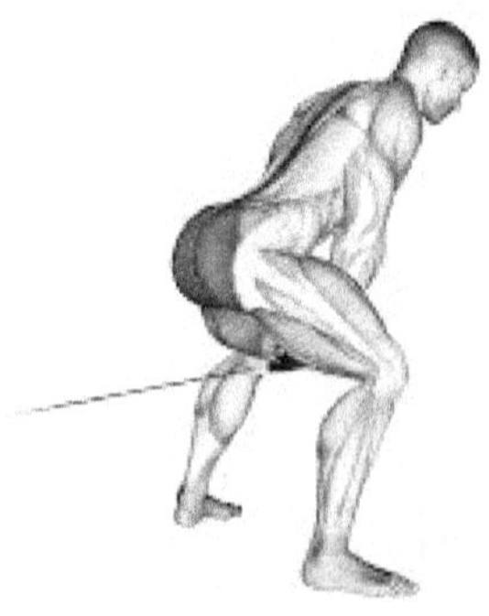

- **Overview**: Cable pull-throughs are a unique glute-focused exercise that utilizes a cable machine for resistance. This movement targets the glutes by encouraging a hip hinge while minimizing lower back strain.

- o **How to Perform**:
    1. Stand facing away from a low cable machine, holding the rope attachment between your legs.
    2. Hinge at the hips, allowing the cable to pull your arms back, feeling the stretch in your hamstrings.
    3. Engage your glutes and return to the starting position by thrusting your hips forward.
- o **Benefits**: Activates the glutes, reinforces proper hip hinging form, and provides an alternative to more traditional exercises like deadlifts.

7. **Kickbacks (Cable or Resistance Band)**

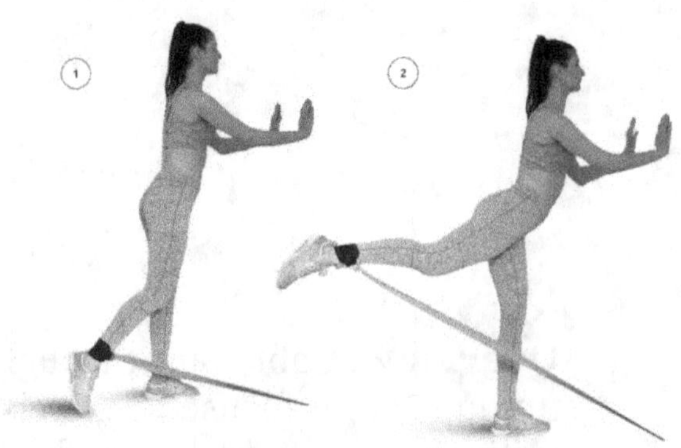

- **Overview**: Glute kickbacks isolate the glutes, specifically the gluteus maximus, providing shape and lift to the backside. This exercise can be performed using a cable machine or resistance bands.
- **How to Perform**:
  1. Attach an ankle strap to a cable machine or loop a resistance band around your legs.
  2. Stand with a slight forward lean, holding onto a support.
  3. Extend one leg straight back, engaging your glute at the top of the movement, then lower with control.
- **Benefits**: Isolates the glutes, improves hip stability, and can be easily modified for different resistance levels.

Tips for Maximizing Glute Engagement

- **Focus on Mind-Muscle Connection**: Concentrate on engaging the glutes with every movement, particularly at the top of each exercise.
- **Prioritize Range of Motion**: Perform each exercise with a full range of motion to activate the glutes thoroughly and increase flexibility.

- **Utilize Progressive Overload**: Gradually increase weight or resistance to continually challenge the muscles and promote growth.
- **Add Variety to Your Routine**: Incorporate a mix of bodyweight, weighted, and resistance band exercises to target the glutes from different angles.

These glute-focused exercises offer a balanced mix of bodyweight, weighted, and resistance-based movements to shape and strengthen the glutes. Consistently practicing these exercises will help you achieve a lifted, toned lower body while enhancing overall lower body strength, balance, and stability.

Tips for Perfect Form: Detailed Cues and Tips to Ensure Maximum Engagement and Prevent Common Mistakes

Proper form is essential in glute-focused exercises to ensure that the target muscles are fully activated and to avoid strain on the lower back, knees, or hips. Below are key cues and tips to maintain perfect form in popular glute exercises:

1. **Hip Thrusts**
   - **Form Cues**: Start with your upper back resting on a bench, feet flat on the ground, and a barbell (or weight) across your hips. Keep your core tight, and drive through your heels as

you lift your hips, focusing on squeezing the glutes at the top.

- o **Common Mistakes**: Avoid arching your back or letting your knees cave inward. Focus on engaging your core throughout to prevent lower back strain.

2. **Glute Bridges**
   - o **Form Cues**: Lie on your back with knees bent, feet hip-width apart. Push through your heels to lift your hips, keeping your back neutral. At the top, squeeze your glutes and hold for a moment before lowering.
   - o **Common Mistakes**: Don't let your hips sag at the top or overextend your lower back. Keep your core tight and avoid pushing through the toes, as this shifts focus away from the glutes.

3. **Step-Ups**
   - o **Form Cues**: Step up onto a bench or sturdy surface with one leg, driving through the heel of the planted foot and engaging the glutes and quads as you lift yourself up.
   - o **Common Mistakes**: Don't rely on momentum or jump up with the other leg. Focus on controlled movements and ensure your knee doesn't move past your toes to protect the joint.

4. **Bulgarian Split Squats**
   - o **Form Cues**: Place one foot behind you on a bench and keep your torso

upright. As you lower into the squat, press through the heel of your front foot and keep your knee aligned with your ankle.

- o **Common Mistakes**: Avoid leaning too far forward or pushing through the back leg. Keep the movement slow and controlled, focusing on activating the glute of the front leg.

5. **Romanian Deadlifts**
   - o **Form Cues**: With a slight bend in your knees, hinge at the hips to lower the weight, keeping your back straight and glutes engaged. As you return to standing, squeeze the glutes at the top.
   - o **Common Mistakes**: Avoid rounding your back or bending the knees too much. Focus on the hip hinge movement rather than a squat, keeping the weight close to your legs throughout.

6. **Kickbacks (Cable or Resistance Band)**
   - o **Form Cues**: Attach the cable or resistance band around your ankle. Stand with a slight forward lean, and extend one leg back, squeezing the glute at the top of the movement.
   - o **Common Mistakes**: Don't swing the leg too high, which can strain the lower back. Keep the motion controlled and focus on the glute contraction at the top.

Importance of Glute Strength: How Stronger Glutes Improve Hip Alignment, Support Posture, and Reduce Lower Back Pain

Strong glutes are critical for maintaining a balanced, stable lower body and for supporting overall functional movement. Here's how glute strength plays a vital role in overall health and fitness:

1. **Improved Hip Alignment**
   - The glutes help stabilize the hips and maintain proper alignment, which is essential for balanced and safe movement in daily activities and workouts. Weak glutes can lead to over-reliance on other muscles, leading to hip misalignment and an increased risk of injury. Strengthening the glutes corrects this imbalance and promotes even weight distribution across the lower body.
2. **Enhanced Posture**
   - Strong glutes play an important role in supporting the lower back and pelvis, which is crucial for good posture. Weak glutes can lead to a forward tilt of the pelvis, causing the lower back to arch excessively, which may lead to poor posture and even back pain over time. When the glutes

are strong and activated, they help stabilize the pelvis and allow for a more upright, aligned spine.

3. **Lower Back Pain Reduction**
   - Weak glutes often lead to overcompensation from the lower back muscles, contributing to strain and discomfort. Strong glutes relieve pressure on the lower back, as they take on a larger share of the workload during activities that involve lifting, bending, and stabilizing the hips. By building glute strength, you're enhancing the body's natural support system, reducing the likelihood of chronic lower back pain.

4. **Increased Power and Athletic Performance**
   - Glute strength is directly linked to improved athletic abilities, particularly in sports or activities that require sprinting, jumping, or lifting. Strong glutes allow for more explosive power, enhancing speed and agility. This benefit translates to everyday activities too, such as climbing stairs, lifting heavy objects, or simply walking with more ease and less fatigue.

5. **Enhanced Core and Pelvic Stability**
   - The glutes are part of the body's core stabilizers and work together with the abdominals and lower back muscles to provide a stable

foundation for movement. When your glutes are strong, they help maintain pelvic stability, which not only improves balance but also reduces the risk of falls and injuries, especially as you age.

6. **Boosted Metabolism and Fat Burning**
   - The glutes are one of the largest muscle groups in the body, meaning they burn a significant amount of calories when activated. Strengthening the glutes can increase your resting metabolic rate and improve your body's fat-burning capacity. Incorporating glute exercises into your routine helps build lean muscle mass, which in turn supports a healthy metabolism and aids in long-term weight management.

This chapter provides readers with a strong foundation in both proper form and understanding of the benefits of glute strength, setting the stage for safe and effective workouts throughout the rest of the book. With detailed form tips and an emphasis on the role of glute strength in overall health, readers are prepared to achieve the sculpted, strong lower body they desire.

Chapter 6: Inner and Outer Thigh Toning

The inner and outer thigh muscles play a key role in lower body stability, balance, and overall leg shape. This chapter focuses on exercises designed to tone and strengthen the adductors (inner thigh muscles) and abductors (outer thigh muscles). By targeting these specific areas, readers will improve hip stability, boost athletic performance, and enhance the aesthetics of the thighs. Here's an in-depth look at key exercises and techniques for sculpting the inner and outer thighs.

Adductor and Abductor Exercises: Moves to Target Inner and Outer Thigh Muscles

1. **Clamshells**

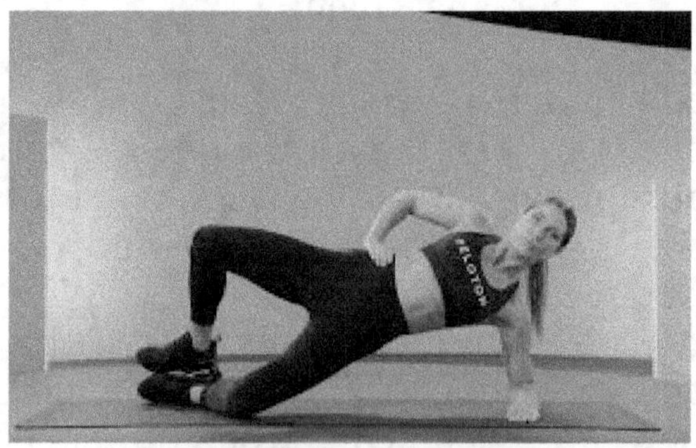

- o **Muscles Worked**: Primarily targets the abductors, particularly the gluteus medius and minimus, along with the outer thighs.

- **How to Do It**: Lie on your side with your knees bent at a 90-degree angle and your feet together. Keeping your feet touching, lift your top knee as high as possible without rotating your pelvis. Slowly lower back to the starting position and repeat.
- **Tips for Effectiveness**: To increase resistance, use a resistance band around your thighs just above your knees. Focus on squeezing the glutes and engaging the outer thighs throughout the movement.

2. **Lateral Band Walks**

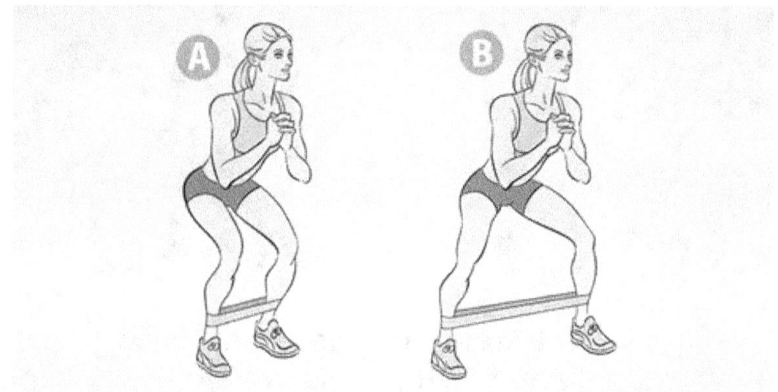

- **Muscles Worked**: Primarily targets the hip abductors and glutes, with secondary activation of the outer thigh muscles.
- **How to Do It**: Place a resistance band around your thighs, just above your knees or around your ankles. Stand with feet hip-width apart, bend

your knees slightly, and take small, controlled steps to the side. Keep your toes pointed forward and avoid leaning your torso.

- o **Tips for Effectiveness**: Keep tension on the band throughout the exercise, and maintain a low, athletic stance. This will ensure consistent activation of the outer thighs and glutes.

3. **Sumo Squats**

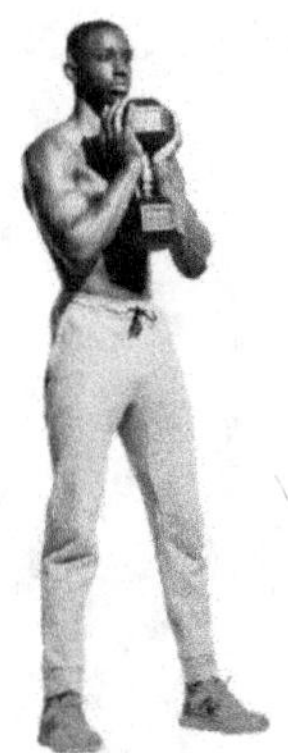
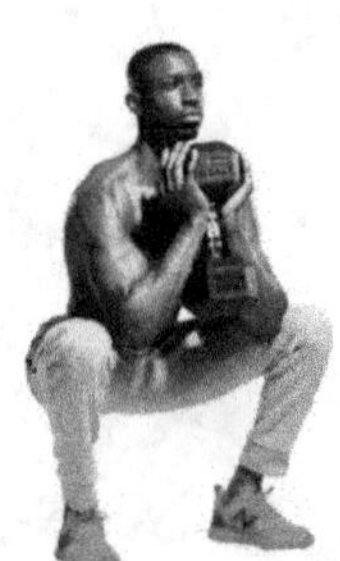

- o **Muscles Worked**: Primarily targets the adductors, glutes, and quadriceps, with secondary activation of the inner thigh muscles.
- o **How to Do It**: Stand with feet wider than shoulder-width apart, with toes pointing slightly outward. Lower into a squat, keeping your chest lifted and back straight. Push through your heels to return to the starting

position, squeezing your glutes and engaging your inner thighs at the top.

- o **Tips for Effectiveness**: Go slow and focus on depth—aim to bring your thighs parallel to the floor. Adding a dumbbell or kettlebell held at chest height can increase resistance and engage the inner thighs even more.

4. **Inner Thigh Leg Raises**

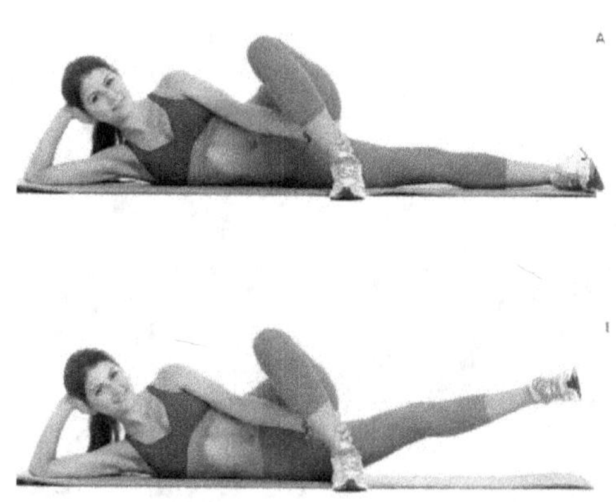

- o **Muscles Worked**: Directly targets the adductors in the inner thighs.
- o **How to Do It**: Lie on your side with your bottom leg extended straight and top leg crossed over. Lift the bottom leg up toward the ceiling, focusing on squeezing the inner thigh, then slowly lower back to the ground.

- Tips for Effectiveness: Perform this move slowly to feel the contraction in the inner thigh. For added resistance, use ankle weights or a resistance band.

5. **Cable Abduction and Adduction**

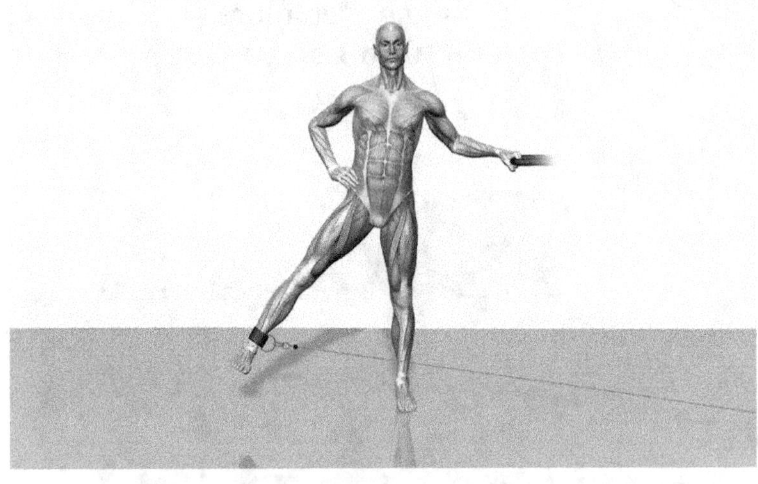

- **Muscles Worked**: Cable abduction targets the abductors and outer thighs, while cable adduction targets the adductors and inner thighs.
- **How to Do It**: For abduction, stand with the cable machine on your side and the ankle attachment around your outer ankle. Lift your leg out to the side, then return it slowly. For adduction, stand with the cable on the opposite side and pull your leg inward across your body.

- o **Tips for Effectiveness**: Keep movements slow and controlled to avoid using momentum. Adjust the cable weight to a level that allows you to maintain form without swaying or compensating with your upper body.

6. **Side Lunges**

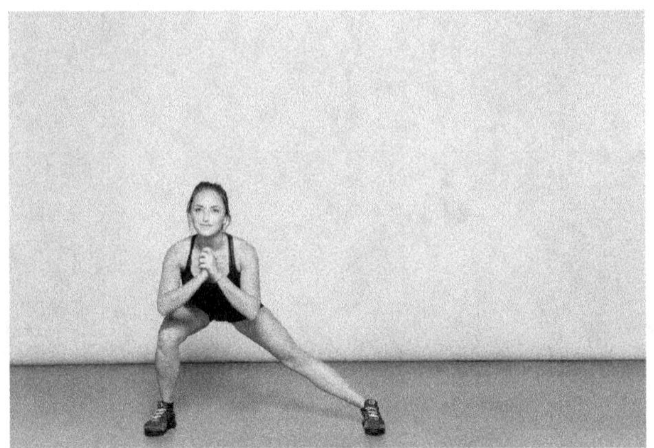

- o **Muscles Worked**: Primarily targets the adductors, abductors, quadriceps, and glutes, with an emphasis on the inner thighs.
- o **How to Do It**: Stand with feet hip-width apart, then step one foot out to the side and lower into a lunge. Keep the other leg straight and your chest lifted as you descend. Push off the bent leg to return to the starting position and repeat on the other side.
- o **Tips for Effectiveness**: Keep your weight in your heel as you lunge to protect your knees and engage the

glutes and inner thighs effectively. Adding weights or a dumbbell can increase the challenge.

7. **Curtsy Lunges**

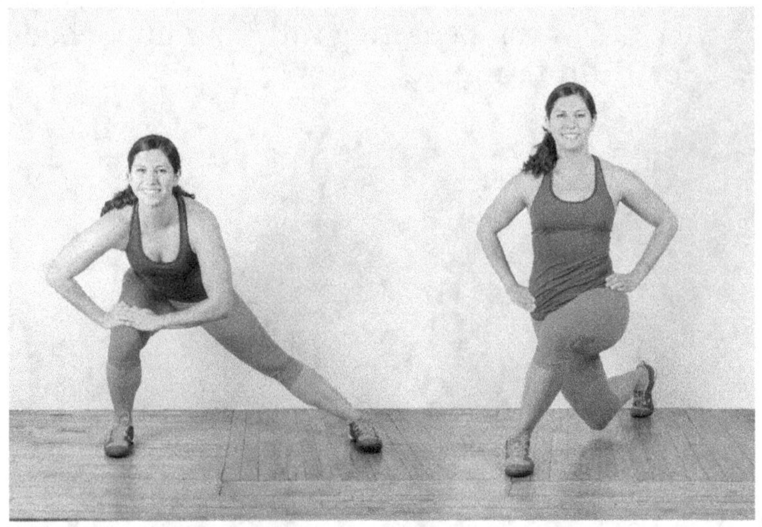

- o **Muscles Worked**: Primarily targets the adductors, glutes, and quadriceps, with secondary emphasis on the inner and outer thighs.
- o **How to Do It**: Stand with feet hip-width apart, then step one leg diagonally behind you and lower into a lunge, keeping your front knee aligned with your front foot. Return to the starting position and repeat on the other side.
- o **Tips for Effectiveness**: Keep your torso upright and avoid leaning forward. Focus on driving through the heel of the front leg to engage the

inner thighs and glutes. Adding dumbbells or a barbell can intensify the exercise.

Why Inner and Outer Thigh Strength Matters

1. **Enhanced Stability and Balance**
   Strong inner and outer thigh muscles help stabilize the pelvis and knees, which is crucial for maintaining balance during dynamic movements like running, jumping, and turning. This stability also supports injury prevention, as weak inner and outer thighs can lead to imbalances and strains on surrounding muscles and joints.
2. **Better Hip Mobility and Function**
   Strengthening the adductors and abductors aids in hip mobility, which is important for activities like climbing stairs, squatting, and bending. Flexible and strong hip muscles improve movement patterns and allow for greater range of motion in the hips and legs.
3. **Sculpted Thighs and Definition**
   Toning the adductors and abductors helps create a leaner, more defined appearance in the thighs, giving the legs a balanced, symmetrical look. These muscles also contribute to the shapely, toned look of the entire lower body.

4. **Injury Prevention and Joint Protection**
   Weak or underdeveloped adductors and abductors can lead to compensations in other muscles, potentially causing knee, hip, and lower back issues. By strengthening these areas, you're providing essential support to the knees and hips, helping prevent strains and injuries during physical activities.
5. **Enhanced Athletic Performance**
   Strong adductors and abductors are key for lateral and multidirectional movement, which is essential in many sports like tennis, soccer, and basketball. Building strength in these muscles boosts agility, speed, and power, enhancing overall athletic ability.

This chapter provides readers with a comprehensive approach to inner and outer thigh toning, incorporating exercises, proper form techniques, and the benefits of strengthening these often-overlooked muscles. With dedication and the right moves, readers will build sculpted, strong, and stable thighs, laying the groundwork for an effective lower body transformation.

Benefits of Toned Thighs: How Strengthening These Muscles Contributes to Overall Leg Shape and Stability

Achieving toned thighs goes beyond aesthetics; strengthening the muscles in the thighs provides a foundation of stability, balance, and functional strength that impacts everyday activities and athletic performance. Here's how toned thighs benefit overall leg shape and stability:

1. **Improved Leg Shape and Definition**
   Strong, toned thigh muscles—particularly the quadriceps, hamstrings, and adductors—add shape and definition to the legs. This definition enhances the natural contours of the thighs, giving them a lean and sculpted appearance. By targeting each muscle group in balanced workouts, you can achieve a proportionate look, adding curves and symmetry that contribute to the classic "legs for days" appearance.

2. **Enhanced Stability and Balance**
   The muscles in the thighs play a crucial role in stabilizing the hips, knees, and ankles. Strengthening the thighs improves stability, which reduces the risk of falls and supports balance during various movements, from walking and running to complex exercises like lunges and squats. This stability is also essential for people with active lifestyles or those who participate in sports, as it provides control over lateral (side-to-side) movements.

3. **Support for the Knees and Hips**
   Toned thighs provide essential support to both the knees and hips, reducing strain on these joints. Strong quadriceps help absorb

shock during high-impact activities, while toned hamstrings provide balance to the knee joint. Balanced thigh muscles alleviate stress on the hips and lower back, as well, which can help prevent injuries associated with weak or imbalanced muscles around these joints.

4. **Increased Functional Strength**
The thigh muscles are heavily involved in daily activities like walking, standing, bending, and lifting. Building strength in these muscles increases overall functional capacity, making everyday tasks feel easier. Activities like climbing stairs, carrying groceries, or lifting objects off the ground require less effort when the thighs are toned and strong.

5. **Better Posture and Alignment**
The thigh muscles, especially the hamstrings and adductors, play a role in maintaining proper posture and alignment. Strengthening the thighs helps prevent inward knee collapse (often caused by weak inner thighs), which can contribute to poor posture and misalignment in the lower body. Toned thighs work with the glutes and core to support an upright posture, reducing the likelihood of lower back pain and enhancing the appearance of a strong, balanced physique.

6. **Improved Athletic Performance**
For those involved in sports or fitness, toned thighs enhance performance by providing power and speed. Strong quads

and hamstrings contribute to explosive movements like sprinting, jumping, and quick directional changes, which are essential in sports like basketball, tennis, and soccer. This power not only improves performance but also reduces fatigue during longer or more demanding activities, as the muscles can handle greater loads efficiently.

7. **Boosted Metabolism and Fat Loss** The thigh muscles are some of the largest muscle groups in the body. Strengthening them through targeted exercises increases muscle mass, which in turn boosts metabolism. A higher metabolic rate means that you burn more calories throughout the day, which aids in overall fat loss, including around the thighs. Regular thigh training helps maintain a leaner physique, contributing to long-term weight management and body composition goals.

8. **Enhanced Mobility and Flexibility** Working on thigh strength often incorporates stretching and mobility exercises, which improve flexibility in the hips, knees, and thighs. Greater flexibility in the thighs reduces stiffness and helps improve range of motion, making it easier to perform dynamic movements without discomfort or risk of strain. Enhanced flexibility in the thighs also translates to smoother, more fluid movement in everyday activities.

The benefits of toned thighs extend far beyond their appearance. Strong, defined thigh muscles are crucial for stability, injury prevention, functional strength, and enhanced physical performance. By dedicating time to thigh workouts, readers can expect to see improvements not only in the shape of their legs but also in overall movement, posture, and metabolic health. As they progress, they'll feel stronger and more confident in their bodies, capable of handling physical demands with ease and enjoying a balanced, resilient lower body.

Resistance Band and Cable Machine Workouts: Using Bands and Cables to Add Intensity to Inner and Outer Thigh Exercises

Resistance bands and cable machines are excellent tools for targeting the inner and outer thigh muscles (adductors and abductors) with greater intensity and precision. These tools provide constant tension, challenging the muscles through the full range of motion, which helps enhance muscle engagement and build strength more effectively.

Here's an in-depth look at how to incorporate resistance bands and cable machines into inner and outer thigh exercises:

1. **Benefits of Resistance Band and Cable Machine Workouts**
    - **Constant Tension**: Resistance bands and cable machines keep tension on the muscles throughout the exercise, which helps with muscle activation and promotes strength gains.
    - **Improved Stability and Control**: Using these tools requires balance and stability, engaging surrounding muscles and the core, which improves control and coordination.
    - **Versatility and Adaptability**: Bands are portable and versatile, while cable machines allow for adjustments in resistance and angle, making them suitable for people at any fitness level.
    - **Reduced Joint Stress**: Both bands and cables offer smooth, controlled resistance, which is easier on the joints than free weights, ideal for those with knee or hip sensitivity.

---

2. **Essential Resistance Band Exercises for Inner and Outer Thighs**
    - **Lateral Band Walks**: Place a resistance band just above the knees or around the ankles and take small side-to-side steps. This movement targets the outer thighs (abductors),

improving hip stability and activating the glutes.

- o **Banded Clamshells**: Lying on your side with a band around your thighs, open and close your top knee while keeping your feet together. Clamshells are excellent for isolating the outer thigh and glute muscles.
- o **Standing Adductor Band Pulls**: Anchor a resistance band to a low point and loop it around one ankle. Stand on one leg, pull your working leg inward against the band's resistance, targeting the inner thighs.
- o **Squat with Lateral Leg Raise**: Start in a squat position with a band around your thighs. Rise up from the squat and lift one leg to the side, alternating legs with each squat. This compound move engages both the inner and outer thighs along with the glutes.

3. **Effective Cable Machine Exercises for Thigh Targeting**
   - o **Cable Abduction**: Attach an ankle strap to the low cable and secure it around your ankle. Standing sideways to the machine, pull your leg outward against the cable's resistance to target the outer thighs.

Keep your torso steady and engage your core for balance.

- o **Cable Adduction**: With the cable anchored low, attach the strap to the ankle of your working leg. Stand sideways and pull your leg inward toward the machine, engaging the inner thigh muscles. This exercise isolates the adductors, strengthening and toning the inner thighs.
- o **Standing Cable Kickback**: Attach the cable to one ankle and, facing the machine, pull your leg straight back. This movement targets the glutes and hamstrings but also activates the outer thighs, contributing to a more defined and lifted lower body.
- o **Cable Side Lunges**: Stand with the cable attached to your outer leg and step to the side into a lunge, pushing against the cable resistance. This exercise works the thighs and glutes while building lateral strength and stability.

4. **Combining Bands and Cables for Maximum Impact**

For an added challenge, some exercises can incorporate both bands and cables to increase muscle activation in the thighs:

- o **Banded Cable Squats**: Place a resistance band around your thighs while holding the cable in front of you or at waist height. Squat down, maintaining tension in the band to engage the outer thighs while the cable provides forward resistance, challenging both the front and sides of the legs.
- o **Cable Clamshells with Band**: With a band around the thighs, use a cable machine for added resistance on one leg during clamshells. This combination intensifies the outer thigh and glute activation, creating a higher level of engagement.

---

5. **Form Tips for Resistance Band and Cable Exercises**
   - o **Focus on Slow, Controlled Movements**: Avoid rushing through the reps. Slow, controlled movements engage the muscle fibers more effectively, especially with resistance bands and cables, where tension is continuous.
   - o **Maintain Core Engagement**: Keeping the core tight prevents compensatory movements, stabilizes the body, and directs the focus to the thighs.

- o **Use Proper Resistance Level**: Start with a lighter band or lower cable weight and gradually increase as strength improves. Excessive resistance can compromise form and reduce effectiveness.
- o **Check Alignment**: When doing abduction or adduction movements, ensure that your knees are aligned with your toes and hips to prevent unnecessary strain.

---

6. Incorporating Resistance Band and Cable Workouts in Your Routine

To make the most of resistance band and cable exercises, consider the following:

- o **Add Variety**: Include different exercises targeting various angles and planes of motion to work all areas of the thighs.
- o **Use as Finishing Moves**: Incorporate these exercises at the end of your workout for a "burnout" effect, thoroughly fatiguing the muscles for maximum toning.
- o **Balance with Bodyweight Exercises**: Combine bands and cables with bodyweight exercises for a balanced routine that improves both muscle strength and endurance.

- **Rest and Recovery**: Because these exercises often work stabilizer muscles intensely, give your body adequate recovery time between sessions.

Using resistance bands and cable machines adds diversity and intensity to inner and outer thigh exercises, helping you achieve stronger, more defined thighs. By incorporating these tools, you'll maximize muscle engagement and accelerate lower body toning, improving balance, stability, and leg shape.

Chapter 7: Core and Hip Flexor Activation

In this chapter, we'll explore the essential connection between a strong core and optimal hip function. While the lower body is often the focus of hip and thigh workouts, the core plays a pivotal role in hip stability, mobility, and overall leg strength. Developing a solid foundation in the core enhances hip movement, supports proper posture, and protects against injuries. Strengthening both the core and hip flexors is a powerful approach to achieving balance, endurance, and control in your lower body workouts.

Core and Hip Connection: The Importance of a Strong Core in Hip Mobility and Stability

1. **Understanding the Core-Hip Relationship**
   - The core isn't just the "abs"—it encompasses the muscles around your torso, including the rectus abdominis, obliques, transverse abdominis, erector spinae, and even the glutes and pelvic floor. These muscles stabilize the spine and pelvis, providing a foundation for lower body movements.
   - Hip flexors, located at the front of the pelvis, work closely with the core to

facilitate movements like lifting the knees and bending at the waist. When these muscles are strong and flexible, they reduce strain on the lower back and enable smooth, controlled hip motions.

2. **Benefits of a Strong Core for Hip Function**

   o **Enhanced Mobility**: A strong core improves range of motion in the hips, allowing for more fluid, controlled leg movements during exercises like squats, lunges, and leg raises.

   o **Injury Prevention**: Weak core muscles can lead to an unstable pelvis and poor posture, increasing the risk of hip, lower back, and knee injuries. By strengthening the core, you create a stable base that reduces strain on the joints and supports healthy alignment.

   o **Improved Athletic Performance**: For athletes, a stable core provides better control during explosive movements such as sprinting, jumping, and cutting. This stability allows for quicker transitions and greater agility in sports and dynamic activities.

   o **Better Balance and Coordination**: The core and hip flexors work together to stabilize the body, particularly during single-leg exercises. Improved core strength enhances balance, coordination, and proprioception, which are crucial for daily activities and athletic performance.

Core Exercises for Hip Stability

Core exercises that target the deep muscles around the spine and pelvis play a crucial role in supporting hip movements. Here's a selection of effective core exercises that specifically aid in hip stability:

1. **Planks**

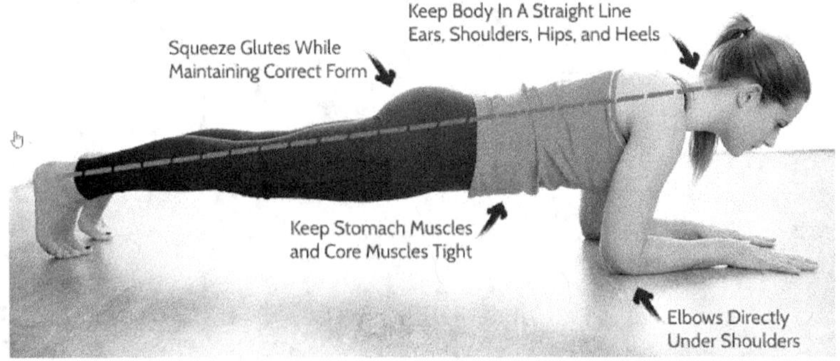

- o Planks are a foundational core exercise that strengthens the entire core region, including the transverse abdominis and obliques, which stabilize the hips. Variations like side planks and forearm planks add further activation to the hip and thigh muscles, enhancing their stability.

- **How to Perform**: Start in a push-up position with elbows directly under the shoulders and hold your body in a straight line from head to heels. Engage the core by pulling the navel toward the spine and maintain the position for as long as possible, focusing on hip and shoulder alignment.

2. **Mountain Climbers**

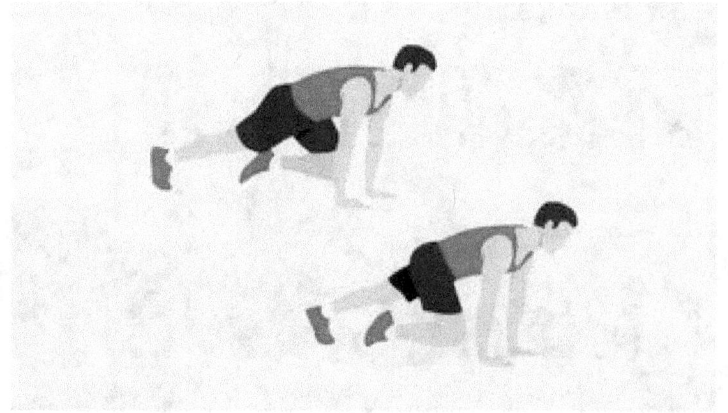

- This dynamic core exercise works both the core and hip flexors while increasing heart rate. It's particularly beneficial for hip flexor endurance, helping to maintain flexibility and strength in the front of the hips.

- o **How to Perform**: Start in a plank position. Drive one knee toward your chest, then quickly switch legs, moving in a controlled, quick-paced motion. Keep your hips steady and avoid sagging or raising them.

3. **Dead Bugs**

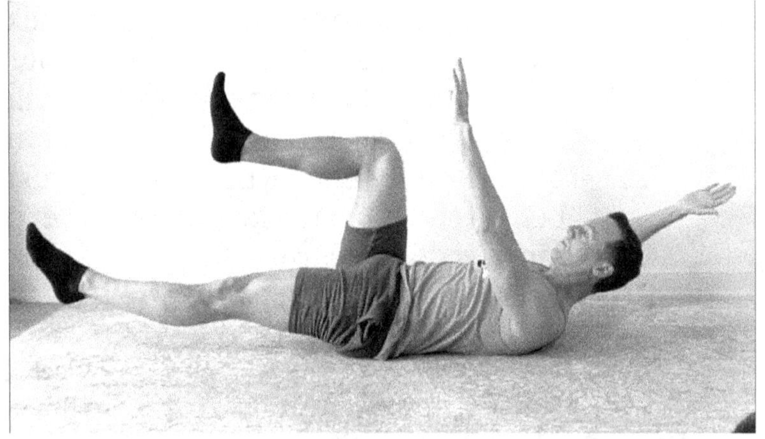

- o Dead bugs are excellent for improving core stability, as they teach you to control movement in the limbs while maintaining a strong, stable core. This exercise also works the hip flexors as you bring your legs toward your torso.
- o **How to Perform**: Lie on your back with arms extended toward the ceiling and legs in a tabletop position. Lower one arm and the opposite leg toward the ground, keeping the core engaged, then

return to the starting position. Repeat on the other side.

4. **Leg Raises**
   - Leg raises engage the lower abdominal muscles and hip flexors, building strength in the core while also activating the muscles around the hips.
   - **How to Perform**: Lie on your back with legs straight. Slowly raise your legs toward the ceiling, keeping them as straight as possible. Lower them back down with control, stopping just before they touch the ground to keep tension on the core.

5. **Russian Twists**

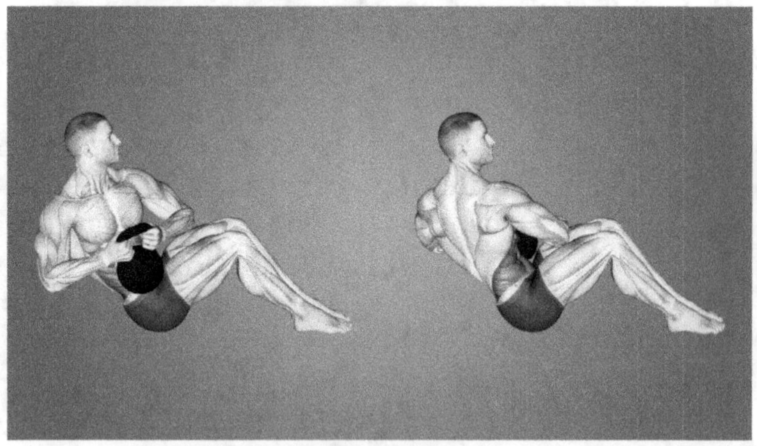

   - This rotational core exercise targets the obliques and stabilizes the hips, which helps with balance and stability in hip-dominant exercises.

- o **How to Perform**: Sit with knees bent, leaning back slightly. Hold a weight (optional) and twist your torso to one side, then the other, engaging the core throughout.

6. **Hip Bridges with Core Focus**

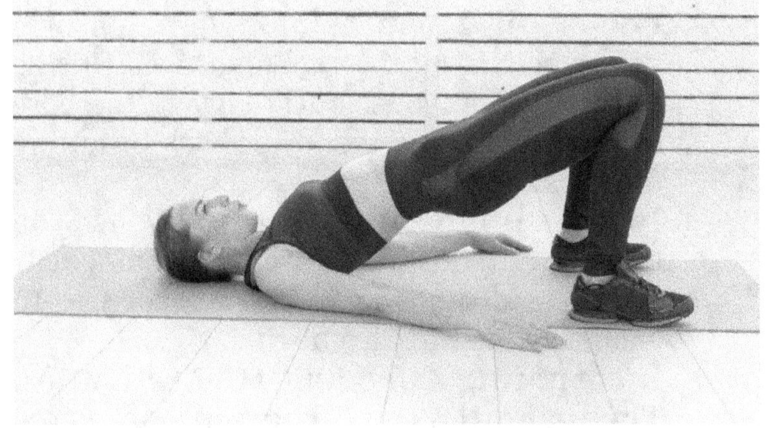

- o Hip bridges target the glutes and hamstrings but also require strong core engagement to keep the hips level and stable.
- o **How to Perform**: Lie on your back with knees bent and feet flat on the floor. Lift your hips off the ground by squeezing your glutes and engaging your core, forming a straight line from shoulders to knees. Hold, then lower with control.

Tips for Integrating Core and Hip Activation into Your Routine

1. **Start with Core Activation**: Beginning your workout with core exercises can "wake up" the core muscles, enhancing their engagement in hip-dominant movements.
2. **Focus on Form**: Proper form ensures you're activating the right muscles. During each exercise, consciously engage the core and avoid arching the lower back or letting the hips tilt.
3. **Increase Difficulty Gradually**: As you build strength, incorporate resistance or longer hold times in your core exercises to challenge the muscles further.
4. **Incorporate Core and Hip Activation Throughout Your Program**: Make core and hip activation exercises a regular part of your routine, performing them at the start of each workout or incorporating them into your warm-up.

By building strength in both the core and hip flexors, you'll gain greater stability and control in lower body movements, reduce injury risks, and achieve better results in your hip and thigh workouts. Developing this foundation will enhance every part of your fitness journey, from lifting heavier weights to improving your balance and coordination in daily activities.

Preventing Tight Hip Flexors: Exercises and Stretches to Balance Hip Flexor Strength and Flexibility

Tight hip flexors are a common issue, particularly for people who spend a lot of time sitting or who engage in high-impact activities like running or cycling. When hip flexors become tight, they can cause discomfort, limit mobility, and increase the risk of injury in both the hips and lower back. To prevent and manage tight hip flexors, it's essential to combine strength and flexibility work with regular stretching. This approach keeps the muscles around the hips balanced, reducing strain on the hip joint and promoting smoother, more fluid movements.

Why Hip Flexor Flexibility Matters

The hip flexors are a group of muscles located at the front of the pelvis and upper thigh, with the primary muscles being the iliopsoas, rectus femoris, and sartorius. These muscles are responsible for lifting the knees toward the chest and stabilizing the pelvis during movement. However, when they're overused or neglected in terms of stretching, they can become shortened and tight, pulling on the pelvis and leading to postural imbalances, limited mobility, and increased risk of lower back pain.

Balancing Hip Flexor Strength and Flexibility

1. **Strengthening the Hip Flexors**: It's important to keep the hip flexors strong to support various lower body movements, particularly in exercises that require lifting or bending the knee. However, this strength should be balanced with flexibility to avoid muscle shortening.
2. **Promoting Flexibility in Hip Flexors**: Regularly stretching the hip flexors improves range of motion, allowing for better form in exercises like squats and lunges. Flexible hip flexors also reduce the risk of pelvic misalignment and can help relieve lower back discomfort caused by tightness in the hips.
3. **Balancing Muscle Groups**: In addition to working the hip flexors, it's important to strengthen the opposing muscle groups, particularly the glutes and hamstrings, which help maintain a balanced pelvis and prevent the hip flexors from becoming overactive.

Effective Exercises and Stretches for Hip Flexor Flexibility

Incorporate the following exercises and stretches into your routine to prevent tightness and maintain a healthy balance between hip flexor strength and flexibility.

Exercises to Strengthen Hip Flexors

1. **Standing Knee Raises**
   - This movement strengthens the hip flexors by focusing on lifting the knee while maintaining core engagement.
   - **How to Perform**: Stand with feet hip-width apart. Lift one knee toward your chest, hold for a second, and then lower back down. Repeat on the other leg. For added resistance, you can perform this exercise with ankle weights.
2. **Seated Leg Lifts**
   - Seated leg lifts target the hip flexors while allowing you to isolate the movement for focused activation.
   - **How to Perform**: Sit on the edge of a chair with feet flat on the floor. Lift one leg straight out in front of you, hold briefly, then lower. Repeat with the other leg. Aim for 10-12 reps per leg.
3. **Mountain Climbers**
   - Mountain climbers are a dynamic exercise that works the hip flexors and core while also providing a cardiovascular benefit.
   - **How to Perform**: Begin in a plank position. Quickly alternate driving one knee toward your chest, then switch legs in a running motion.

Keep the core engaged and hips level throughout.

Stretches to Improve Hip Flexor Flexibility

1. **Lunge Stretch (Low Lunge)**
   - This stretch deeply opens up the hip flexors, targeting the iliopsoas and quadriceps.
   - **How to Perform**: Step one foot forward into a lunge position and lower the back knee to the floor. Shift your weight forward, allowing the hips to sink. Hold for 20-30 seconds, then switch sides. For a deeper stretch, reach both arms overhead and lean slightly back.
2. **Pigeon Pose**
   - Pigeon pose is a yoga stretch that targets the hip flexors and external hip rotators.
   - **How to Perform**: Start in a plank position. Bring your right knee forward and place it behind your right wrist, allowing the left leg to stretch out behind you. Lower your body over the front leg, keeping the hips square. Hold for 30 seconds to 1 minute, then switch sides.
3. **Hip Flexor and Quad Stretch**

- o This combination stretch is especially effective after lower body workouts to release tightness.
  - o **How to Perform**: In a kneeling position, bring one foot up behind you, holding it with the same-side hand (similar to a quadriceps stretch). Lean forward slightly with the hips to deepen the stretch. Hold for 20-30 seconds, then switch sides.

4. **Crescent Lunge Stretch**
   - o A dynamic version of the lunge stretch that engages the hip flexors through movement.
   - o **How to Perform**: Step into a lunge position with the right leg forward. Reach both arms overhead, then push the left hip forward slightly. Hold for a moment, release, and repeat on the other side.

5. **Butterfly Stretch with Forward Lean**
   - o While this stretch primarily targets the inner thighs, the forward lean helps release tension in the hip flexors.
   - o **How to Perform**: Sit with the soles of your feet together and knees bent outward. Gently press your knees toward the floor while leaning forward slightly to feel a stretch in the hip region.

Preventing Tightness: Tips for Consistent Hip Flexor Maintenance

1. **Incorporate Daily Stretching**: Stretching for even a few minutes daily can prevent the hip flexors from becoming tight and overworked, especially if you spend long periods sitting.
2. **Warm Up Before Exercise**: A dynamic warm-up that includes gentle hip-openers, like leg swings and lunges, prepares the hip flexors for activity and reduces the chance of strain.
3. **Focus on Form**: During strength exercises that engage the hip flexors, pay attention to your form. Proper alignment and muscle engagement prevent overuse and promote balanced muscle activation.
4. **Balance with Glute and Core Strengthening**: Since the glutes and core play a crucial role in supporting the hips, including glute bridges, planks, and other core-focused exercises can prevent the hip flexors from compensating or becoming overly tight.

By incorporating these exercises and stretches, you'll keep your hip flexors flexible and strong, which not only enhances your performance in lower body workouts but also supports overall posture, mobility, and balance.

Part 3: Building Your Lower Body Routine

Chapter 8: Designing Your Workout Plan

Creating an effective lower body workout routine requires understanding how to balance your training days, gradually increase intensity, and allow for proper recovery. This chapter guides you through structuring a well-rounded fitness plan focused on hip, thigh, and overall leg strength, helping you achieve your goals whether they include toning, strength, or power.

How to Structure Your Week

1. **Balancing Lower Body and Upper Body Days**
   - To avoid overtraining any one area, it's important to plan dedicated lower body days as part of your weekly routine. A typical weekly structure might include two to three lower body workouts, two upper body workouts, and at least one cardio or full-body conditioning day.
   - Example Routine:
     - **Day 1**: Lower Body Focus
     - **Day 2**: Upper Body Strength
     - **Day 3**: Cardio or Active Recovery
     - **Day 4**: Lower Body Focus
     - **Day 5**: Upper Body Endurance

- **Day 6**: Lower Body Power Moves or Core + Lower Body
- **Day** 7: Rest or Gentle Stretching

2. Incorporating Cardio for Fat Burning and Endurance

- Cardio sessions, especially low-impact forms like cycling or incline walking, can support lower body goals by improving endurance without overly straining the legs. Including cardio also helps create a calorie deficit, aiding in fat loss.

3. Total Body and Core Workouts for Balance

- In addition to lower body-specific workouts, total body strength or core-focused days promote balance, core stability, and functional strength. This approach ensures your body develops harmoniously, preventing injury and enhancing performance.

Reps, Sets, and Progressions

1. Understanding Reps and Sets

- **Beginners**: Focus on lower rep ranges (8-10 reps) with lighter weights or just body weight to learn proper form.

- **Intermediate**: Increase reps to 10-15 per set, and add resistance with weights or bands for enhanced muscle engagement and strength gains.
- **Advanced**: For those seeking to maximize strength and muscle growth, aim for 6-8 reps per set with heavier weights or increase reps for endurance-focused routines.

2. **Choosing the Right Rep Range Based on Goals**
   - **Strength and Power**: Lower reps (6-8) with heavier weights help build strength and increase muscle size.
   - **Endurance and Tone**: Higher reps (15-20) with lighter weights or body weight promote muscular endurance and toning.
   - **Balance of Both**: Moderate reps (10-12) at a challenging weight will enhance both strength and endurance.

3. **Progressing Your Workouts**
   - As your body adapts, it's important to increase the intensity of your workouts to continue seeing progress. You can do this by:
     - **Increasing Resistance**: Gradually add weight to your exercises.
     - **Adding Reps or Sets**: For endurance, add extra reps or

sets to increase the volume of your workout.

- **Decreasing Rest Time**: Shortening rest between sets can increase the workout's intensity, challenging your endurance and cardiovascular fitness.
- **Incorporating Advanced Variations**: Progress to more complex exercises, such as moving from bodyweight lunges to weighted or plyometric lunges, to push your limits further.

Rest and Recovery

1. **Why Recovery Days Are Essential**
   - Recovery is crucial to allow muscles to repair and grow. Overworking the legs without rest can lead to injury, fatigue, and slower progress. Aim for at least one to two days per week dedicated to full recovery or active recovery activities like gentle walking or yoga.
2. **Foam Rolling and Muscle Release**
   - Foam rolling is a form of self-myofascial release that helps alleviate muscle tightness, improve flexibility, and promote blood flow. Focus on

areas such as the quads, hamstrings, glutes, and calves after each lower body session.

- o **How to Foam Roll**: Roll slowly over each muscle group for 20-30 seconds, pausing on tight or sore spots. For deeper release, try applying more pressure by lifting one leg at a time off the roller.

3. **Importance of Stretching and Mobility Work**

- o Stretching after workouts helps release muscle tension, improve flexibility, and reduce muscle soreness. Focus on dynamic stretching (such as leg swings) before workouts and static stretching (like hamstring stretches) after workouts.
- o Mobility exercises such as hip circles and leg swings keep your joints healthy and promote a full range of motion, essential for lower body strength and injury prevention.

4. **Sleep and Nutrition for Muscle Growth and Repair**

- o Quality sleep and a balanced diet rich in protein, vitamins, and minerals are vital for muscle recovery and growth. Aim for 7-9 hours of sleep and include nutrient-dense foods that support muscle repair, such as lean proteins, leafy greens, and whole grains.

By following these guidelines, you'll be able to design a balanced, progressive, and effective lower body workout routine that leads to strength, tone, and functional fitness in the hips, thighs, and glutes. Whether you're a beginner or an advanced fitness enthusiast, this structured approach will guide you toward achieving the lower body transformation you desire.

Chapter 9: Beginner Routines

Starting a new fitness journey can be both exciting and challenging, especially when focusing on specific areas like the hips, thighs, and glutes. Chapter 9 is designed to ease beginners into lower body training, offering straightforward routines that build foundational strength and confidence. Through bodyweight exercises and light resistance, readers will learn to engage core muscle groups, master basic moves, and establish a strong foundation for future progress.

Quick Start Lower Body Workouts

1. **Introduction to Beginner-Friendly Workouts**
   o These routines use minimal equipment, making them perfect for home or gym environments. The emphasis is on bodyweight exercises,

resistance bands, and light dumbbells, ensuring each workout is accessible for those just starting out.

- o The goal is to introduce essential movement patterns like squats, lunges, and bridges, allowing beginners to build muscle awareness and develop good form before moving on to more challenging variations.

2. **Sample Quick Start Workouts**
    - o **Workout A: Bodyweight Basics**
        - **Bodyweight Squats**: 3 sets of 10-12 reps
        - **Glute Bridges**: 3 sets of 10-12 reps
        - **Standing Calf Raises**: 3 sets of 12-15 reps
        - **Lateral Leg Raises**: 2 sets of 10-12 reps per leg
        - **Cooldown**: Gentle hamstring and quad stretches (30 seconds each side)
    - o **Workout B: Light Resistance with Bands**
        - **Banded Squats**: 3 sets of 10-12 reps
        - **Side-Step Band Walks**: 2 sets of 10 steps per side
        - **Lunges**: 3 sets of 8-10 reps per leg (bodyweight or with light dumbbells)
        - **Donkey Kicks**: 2 sets of 10 reps per leg

- **Cooldown**: Hip flexor and glute stretches (30 seconds each side)

3. **Using Minimal Equipment to Maximize Results**
   - With a simple resistance band or light dumbbells, beginners can add just enough resistance to feel the muscles work harder without overloading their joints. Light equipment allows gradual progression and builds the confidence needed to transition to more intense routines.

Progressing with Confidence

1. **Recognizing Signs of Strength Improvement**
   - As beginners gain strength and endurance, they may notice improvements in balance, mobility, and muscle tone. These changes signify progress and readiness to increase workout intensity or try more complex moves.
   - Tips for noticing progress include tracking reps and sets, noting improvements in form, and keeping a workout journal to celebrate small wins, like completing extra reps or using a slightly heavier weight.

2. **Gradually Increasing Workout Intensity**
   - For continued growth, add one small progression per workout. Beginners can:
     - **Increase Reps**: If completing 10 reps feels manageable, aim for 12-15 reps in the next session.
     - **Add Resistance**: Transition from bodyweight to light weights or bands as strength builds.
     - **Incorporate Tempo Changes**: Slowing down each rep (e.g., a 3-second descent in squats) increases time under tension, helping to build endurance and muscle control.
     - **Add Extra Sets**: Move from 2 sets to 3 or 4 as stamina and confidence increase.
3. **Maintaining Motivation and Positive Mindset**
   - Progress may feel gradual, but maintaining consistency is key to long-term success. Set realistic, achievable milestones, such as completing workouts twice a week for a month or mastering a specific exercise.
   - Use reminders and motivational techniques to keep going even when results aren't immediately visible.

Focus on the positive energy, improved mobility, and strength gains achieved with each session.

- Remember that every bit of progress counts, and building a foundation of strength now prepares you for more advanced routines in the future.

Chapter 10: Intermediate Routines

As readers progress in their fitness journey, Chapter 10 introduces intermediate routines to challenge and enhance lower body strength, endurance, and stability. These routines incorporate weights, dynamic movements, and more complex exercise variations to encourage muscle growth, improve power, and build endurance. Designed for those with a foundation in basic lower body exercises, these routines take leg and glute training to the next level, pushing readers to achieve a stronger, more defined lower body.

Increasing Strength and Endurance

1. **Transitioning from Beginner to Intermediate Workouts**
   - For readers who have built a foundation with beginner routines, intermediate workouts introduce heavier weights, more volume, and higher intensity movements. These changes stimulate further muscle development and improve muscular endurance.
   - Intermediate routines include weighted exercises, like squats with barbells or kettlebells, and incorporate more challenging multi-

muscle moves, like Bulgarian split squats and reverse lunges.

2. **Key Benefits of Intermediate Routines**
    - **Enhanced Strength and Definition**: Adding resistance and dynamic movements helps shape and tone muscles, especially in the glutes, quads, and hamstrings.
    - **Improved Endurance**: Longer sets and higher repetitions challenge the muscles to work harder, helping readers sustain physical activity for extended periods.
    - **Increased Caloric Burn**: Higher-intensity moves elevate heart rate, promoting calorie burn and aiding in fat loss, contributing to a leaner physique.

Sample Intermediate Workouts

1. **Workout A: Weighted Leg and Glute Power Routine**
    - This workout builds power and strength in the glutes, quads, and hamstrings, with an emphasis on controlled, weighted movements to improve form and endurance.
    - **Goblet Squats**: 3 sets of 12 reps (holding a heavy dumbbell or kettlebell)

- o **Bulgarian Split Squats**: 3 sets of 10 reps per leg (with dumbbells)
  - o **Deadlifts**: 3 sets of 12 reps (using a barbell or kettlebells for hamstring focus)
  - o **Kettlebell Swings**: 3 sets of 15 reps (to engage glutes and build power)
  - o **Cooldown**: Foam rolling and hamstring, quad, and glute stretches (30 seconds each)

2. **Workout B: Dynamic Endurance and Plyometric Routine**
  - o Designed to improve endurance and boost strength, this workout includes explosive plyometric moves, which enhance power and speed, and can be adjusted to suit gym or home settings.
  - o **Lateral Step-Ups with Dumbbells**: 3 sets of 12 reps per leg
  - o **Reverse Lunges**: 3 sets of 12 reps per leg (holding dumbbells)
  - o **Plyometric Jump Squats**: 3 sets of 15 reps (bodyweight, focusing on explosive power)
  - o **Single-Leg Deadlift with Dumbbell**: 3 sets of 10 reps per leg (to improve balance and hamstring strength)
  - o **Cooldown**: Dynamic stretching and hip openers to relax and improve flexibility

Tips for Increasing Weight and Intensity Safely

1. **Progress Gradually**
   - As strength improves, increase weights in small increments—by about 5-10% at a time—rather than making drastic changes. Maintaining form is key to preventing injuries.
2. **Focus on Form Over Speed**
   - Prioritize smooth, controlled movements to fully activate the muscles and prevent strain. Intermediate routines encourage higher reps with challenging weight, so maintaining form is essential for effective progress.
3. **Introduce Supersets and Circuit Training**
   - For a boost in endurance and to increase the intensity of the workouts, consider combining exercises into supersets (two exercises performed back-to-back) or circuits, with minimal rest between moves. This not only raises the challenge but also enhances cardiovascular fitness and endurance.

Staying Motivated and Tracking Progress

1. **Set Milestones and Celebrate Achievements**
   - Establish intermediate goals, such as achieving a certain squat weight or completing a full routine without stopping. Celebrate milestones to stay motivated and enjoy the sense of progress.
2. **Regularly Track Performance and Make Adjustments**
   - Keep track of weights, reps, and sets in a workout journal. This allows readers to monitor their progress and make adjustments as strength and endurance improve. Progress tracking also offers motivation on days when results feel gradual.
3. **Focus on the Benefits Beyond Physical Change**
   - Remember that strength training improves energy, stability, posture, and overall well-being. These benefits add value to the workout journey and reinforce the commitment to regular exercise.

Supersets and Circuits

In this section, readers are introduced to the power of supersets and circuit training—two workout structures that combine multiple exercises to amplify strength, enhance endurance, and maximize calorie burn. These methods are ideal for intermediate and advanced readers seeking to intensify their workouts, cut down on workout time, and boost cardiovascular fitness without sacrificing strength gains.

Supersets: What They Are and How They Work

A superset combines two exercises performed back-to-back with minimal rest in between. The two exercises can target the same muscle group (e.g., squats and lunges for the quads) or different muscle groups (e.g., deadlifts for hamstrings followed by abductor exercises). Supersets are an efficient way to add intensity to a routine, making it possible to get more work done in less time while challenging muscles to adapt to higher workloads.

- **Types of Supersets:**
  - **Same Muscle Group Superset**: Works one muscle group with two different exercises, increasing fatigue and muscle engagement.
    - Example: Goblet squats followed by jump squats (both target the quadriceps and glutes)
  - **Opposing Muscle Group Superset**: Works opposite muscle

groups, allowing one to rest while the other is engaged.

- Example: Hamstring curls paired with leg extensions (hamstrings vs. quadriceps)
  - **Upper and Lower Body Superset**: Combines upper and lower body moves for a full-body workout, ideal for busy schedules.
    - Example: Dumbbell lunges followed by shoulder presses (legs and shoulders)
- **Benefits of Supersets**:
  - **Efficient and Time-Saving**: By minimizing rest, supersets allow readers to complete workouts in less time without sacrificing intensity.
  - **Improved Muscle Endurance**: Supersets keep muscles engaged for longer, leading to better endurance over time.
  - **Elevated Caloric Burn**: The continuous movement keeps heart rate elevated, boosting calorie burn and fat loss.

Sample Superset Workout for Legs and Glutes

1. **Goblet Squats**: 3 sets of 12 reps (holding a dumbbell or kettlebell)

2. **Jump Squats**: 3 sets of 15 reps (bodyweight only for explosive power)

- Rest for 60-90 seconds, then repeat.

3. **Deadlifts**: 3 sets of 10 reps (using a barbell or dumbbells)
4. **Hamstring Curls**: 3 sets of 12 reps (on a machine or with resistance bands)

- Rest for 60-90 seconds, then repeat.

5. **Lateral Band Walks**: 3 sets of 20 steps per side
6. **Step-Ups**: 3 sets of 12 reps per leg (holding dumbbells)

Circuit Training: Full Lower Body Engagement

Circuit training consists of a series of exercises performed one after another with minimal rest, targeting different muscle groups to keep the body engaged. Each circuit can include a mix of lower body, core, and cardio-based moves, delivering a well-rounded workout that improves strength, cardiovascular fitness, and endurance. Circuit training is ideal for boosting metabolic rate and offers a time-efficient way to hit multiple muscle groups in a single session.

- **Benefits of Circuit Training**:

- o **High Calorie Burn**: Circuits elevate the heart rate and maintain it throughout the workout, maximizing calorie burn.
- o **Full-Body Conditioning**: With circuits, multiple muscle groups are trained in one session, leading to a balanced, full-body workout.
- o **Improved Cardiovascular Fitness**: Short rest intervals provide a cardio effect, making circuits an excellent choice for both strength and endurance.

Sample Lower Body Circuit Routine

1. **Kettlebell Swings**: 45 seconds (for glutes and hamstrings)
2. **Reverse Lunges with Dumbbells**: 45 seconds per leg
3. **Mountain Climbers**: 45 seconds (for core and cardio boost)
4. **Lateral Band Walks**: 45 seconds per side
5. **Glute Bridges**: 45 seconds

- Rest for 1-2 minutes after completing all exercises, then repeat for 2-3 rounds.

Tips for Incorporating Supersets and Circuits

1. **Start Slow**: For those new to these methods, start with 1-2 supersets or a simple 2-exercise circuit and gradually build up to more challenging combinations.
2. **Monitor Form**: It's tempting to rush through supersets and circuits, but maintaining form is crucial to prevent injuries and fully engage target muscles.
3. **Adjust Intensity as Needed**: As fitness improves, increase weights or add another exercise to each superset or circuit for continued progression.

Supersets and circuits offer a powerful way to take lower body training to new heights, delivering strength, endurance, and cardio benefits in a single workout. By incorporating these techniques, readers can expect to experience faster muscle growth, improved definition, and increased stamina, all while staying efficient with their workout time. This structured approach will enable readers to feel stronger, more agile, and more confident in every step of their fitness journey.

Chapter 11: Advanced Routines

Power and Performance-Based Training

In this chapter, readers are introduced to advanced lower body routines designed to maximize power, agility, and overall athletic performance. These workouts are ideal for those with a solid fitness foundation who are ready to push their limits with heavier weights, plyometric exercises, and explosive movements. Power and performance-based training is essential for developing muscle strength, increasing endurance, and boosting speed, balance, and coordination.

The Role of Power Training in Lower Body Fitness

Power training emphasizes explosive movements, which engage both fast-twitch muscle fibers and enhance muscular power. These routines help develop quick, forceful muscle contractions that are beneficial for athletic performance and everyday activities, like lifting or sprinting. By adding high-intensity exercises, readers will improve not only the strength but also the functionality of their lower body, preparing them for more challenging activities.

- **Benefits of Power and Performance Training:**

o **Increased Muscular Power**: Helps muscles generate more force, improving athletic abilities like jumping and sprinting.
o **Enhanced Speed and Agility**: Fast-twitch muscle activation leads to quicker movements and better reflexes.
o **Improved Coordination and Balance**: High-intensity exercises challenge the body's stability, enhancing balance and core strength.

Key Components of Power-Based Lower Body Workouts

1. **Plyometrics**: Explosive exercises that use body weight to develop strength, speed, and power.
   o Examples: Box jumps, jump squats, and broad jumps.
2. **Heavier Weights and Low Reps**: Advanced lifters benefit from heavy weights with low reps, focusing on strength and muscle endurance.
   o Examples: Heavy barbell squats, deadlifts, and lunges.
3. **Tempo and Rest Intervals**: By altering tempo (how fast or slow exercises are performed) and incorporating short rest intervals, these routines increase intensity.

- o Example: Performing squats with a slow descent and explosive rise to target power.
4. **Combination of Strength and Cardio**: High-intensity moves paired with strength exercises raise the heart rate, supporting cardiovascular health and endurance.

Sample Power and Performance-Based Lower Body Routine

This routine combines strength and plyometrics to challenge all aspects of lower body fitness. Perform each set with a focus on explosive power and good form.

Warm-Up: 5-10 minutes of dynamic stretching and light cardio (e.g., high knees, butt kicks)

1. **Heavy Barbell Squats**: 4 sets of 6 reps
   - o Focus on using a weight that challenges the muscles but allows for controlled, deep squats.
2. **Box Jumps**: 4 sets of 8 reps
   - o Land softly on each jump to minimize impact and build explosive power.
3. **Bulgarian Split Squats with Dumbbells**: 3 sets of 8 reps per leg
   - o Engage the core for balance and control, and use a moderate to heavy weight for increased intensity.

4. **Deadlifts**: 4 sets of 6 reps
   - Use a challenging weight and focus on proper hip hinge movement to maximize hamstring and glute activation.
5. **Broad Jumps**: 3 sets of 10 reps
   - Perform with maximum effort, aiming for a long and controlled landing.
6. **Weighted Step-Ups**: 3 sets of 10 reps per leg
   - Use a high bench or box to increase the range of motion and maximize glute engagement.

Cool-Down: Finish with 5-10 minutes of static stretching, focusing on hamstrings, quads, glutes, and hip flexors.

Advanced Techniques for Greater Results

1. **Eccentric Training**: Slow down the lowering phase of each exercise to increase muscle tension and maximize strength gains.
   - Example: Lower slowly in a squat for 3-4 seconds, then explode up.
2. **Supersets with Explosive Moves**: Pair a heavy strength exercise with a plyometric move for more intensity.
   - Example: Pair heavy squats with jump squats for a powerful

combination that pushes the muscles to the limit.

3. **Progressive Overload**: Gradually increase the weight, reps, or intensity to keep challenging muscles.
    o This approach ensures continuous improvement and prevents plateaus.

Tips for Advanced Power Training

- **Prioritize Recovery**: Advanced training can be hard on muscles, so be mindful of rest days and incorporate recovery practices like foam rolling and stretching.
- **Listen to Your Body**: Power workouts require high energy and focus; avoid pushing through pain, and prioritize quality over quantity.
- **Stay Consistent with Form**: Technique is critical with heavy weights and plyometrics to avoid injury and maximize results.

Power and performance-based training offers a way to take lower body workouts to the next level, building strength, speed, and agility while enhancing functional fitness. By following these advanced routines, readers will develop powerful, resilient legs that perform exceptionally in workouts and everyday life alike, helping them feel confident, capable, and unstoppable in their fitness journey.

Targeted Workouts for Specific Goals

In this section, readers will find tailored workout programs designed to achieve distinct lower body fitness goals, whether they're aiming to build muscle, enhance endurance, or improve muscle definition. Each program is structured with exercises and techniques that specifically address the desired outcome, ensuring efficient and effective progress toward individual fitness aspirations.

---

1. Muscle-Building Program

This program focuses on increasing lower body muscle size and strength through hypertrophy training, which involves moderate to heavy weights and higher volumes (sets and reps). Compound movements are emphasized for maximum muscle engagement, and the program includes isolation exercises to target specific muscles for balanced growth.

Key Elements of the Muscle-Building Program:

- **Moderate to Heavy Weights**: Lift weights that are challenging yet manageable with proper form.

- **Higher Volume**: 3-5 sets of 8-12 reps per exercise.
- **Slow, Controlled Movements**: Maximize muscle tension by focusing on the eccentric (lowering) phase of each lift.

Sample Muscle-Building Workout:

1. **Barbell Squats**: 4 sets of 8-10 reps
2. **Deadlifts**: 4 sets of 8 reps
3. **Bulgarian Split Squats**: 3 sets of 10 reps per leg
4. **Leg Press**: 3 sets of 10-12 reps
5. **Calf Raises**: 4 sets of 15 reps

Progression Tips:

- **Increase Weights Gradually**: Aim to add 5-10% more weight every 1-2 weeks.
- **Focus on Muscle Activation**: Engage the target muscles throughout each rep to stimulate growth.

2. Endurance-Building Program

This program is designed to improve muscular endurance, enabling the legs to sustain prolonged physical activities without fatigue. Endurance training generally involves lighter weights, higher reps, and shorter rest intervals. The workout incorporates dynamic movements to build stamina and improve cardiovascular fitness.

Key Elements of the Endurance-Building Program:

- **High Repetitions**: 12-20 reps per set to build endurance.
- **Minimal Rest**: Short rest periods (30-45 seconds) to maintain an elevated heart rate.
- **Functional Movements**: Exercises that mimic real-life activities, such as step-ups or lunges.

Sample Endurance Workout:

1. **Walking Lunges**: 3 sets of 15-20 reps per leg
2. **Step-Ups**: 4 sets of 20 reps per leg
3. **Bodyweight Squats**: 3 sets of 25 reps
4. **Single-Leg Romanian Deadlifts**: 3 sets of 15 reps per leg
5. **High-Knee Jog in Place**: 3 sets of 60 seconds

Progression Tips:

- **Increase Reps**: Gradually add more reps or sets as endurance improves.
- **Reduce Rest Time**: Aim to complete the workout with shorter breaks to build stamina.

3. Definition-Focused Program

This program emphasizes exercises and training techniques to enhance muscle definition, aiming for a lean, sculpted look in the lower body. Circuit-style workouts, supersets, and high-intensity intervals combine to reduce body fat while toning the legs. The workouts incorporate both strength and cardio elements for maximum calorie burn and muscle shaping.

Key Elements of the Definition-Focused Program:

- **Supersets and Circuits**: Combine exercises back-to-back to maintain intensity and engage multiple muscle groups.
- **Moderate Weights, Moderate Reps**: Generally, 3-4 sets of 10-15 reps.
- **High-Intensity Intervals**: Incorporate short bursts of cardio to keep the heart rate elevated, increasing fat burn.

Sample Definition Workout:

1. **Superset**:
   o Goblet Squats: 3 sets of 12 reps
   o Jump Squats: 3 sets of 15 reps
2. **Superset**:
   o Dumbbell Lunges: 3 sets of 10 reps per leg
   o Lateral Band Walks: 3 sets of 20 steps per side

3. **Circuit**:
   - Calf Raises: 3 sets of 15 reps
   - Box Jumps: 3 sets of 10 reps
   - Mountain Climbers: 3 sets of 30 seconds

Progression Tips:

- **Increase Intensity**: Reduce rest between sets and circuits to keep the heart rate up.
- **Add Cardio Intervals**: Finish with a short, high-intensity cardio blast like sprinting to enhance fat burn.

These targeted programs enable readers to tailor their workouts to align with their personal fitness goals, empowering them to choose routines that suit their needs, whether they want to build muscle, improve stamina, or achieve lean definition in the hips and thighs. By following these structured workouts, readers will see targeted progress in their lower body fitness journey, achieving strength, endurance, or a sculpted physique with purpose and focus.

Part 4: Supporting Your Workouts with Nutrition and Lifestyle

Chapter 12: Nutrition for a Strong and Toned Lower Body

Overview: This chapter highlights the essential role of nutrition in building a strong, toned lower body. It provides readers with practical guidance on pre- and post-workout meal choices, nutrients that support muscle recovery and growth, and the impact of hydration. Proper nutrition is the foundation for fueling workouts, enhancing performance, and aiding recovery, all of which contribute to achieving defined, powerful legs.

Pre- and Post-Workout Nutrition: Fueling for Optimal Energy and Recovery

The right nutrition around workout times can make a significant difference in energy levels, endurance, and how well the body recovers afterward. This section explains why timing, macronutrient balance, and food choices matter.

- **Pre-Workout Nutrition**: Consuming a balanced meal before exercising can provide the energy needed for intense lower body workouts.
  - **Carbohydrates**: Complex carbs like oats, whole grains, and fruits supply sustained energy, preventing fatigue during workouts.
  - **Protein**: Protein sources such as Greek yogurt, eggs, or lean meats support muscle retention and provide amino acids that help prepare muscles for exercise.

- o **Timing**: Aim to eat a pre-workout meal 1-2 hours before exercising. A lighter snack can be eaten 30-45 minutes before a workout if short on time.
- **Post-Workout Nutrition**: After exercising, the body requires nutrients to repair muscle fibers and replenish glycogen (energy stores).
  - o **Protein for Recovery**: Including protein in post-workout meals is essential for muscle repair and growth. Aim for 20-30 grams of protein from sources like chicken, fish, eggs, or plant-based proteins.
  - o **Carbs for Replenishment**: Carbs are needed to restore glycogen levels, which supports recovery and prepares the body for the next workout. Pairing protein with carbs like sweet potatoes, rice, or quinoa is ideal.
  - o **Timing**: Try to eat within 30-60 minutes post-workout to maximize recovery.

This section includes sample meal ideas and snacks that combine protein and carbs, providing practical options for readers to fuel effectively around their workouts.

Key Nutrients for Lower Body Muscle Support

To build and maintain strong, toned muscles in the hips, thighs, and glutes, specific nutrients play vital roles in supporting muscle function, growth, and recovery.

- **Protein**: Critical for muscle repair and growth, protein provides the building blocks (amino acids) that support muscle strength and recovery.
    - **Sources**: Lean meats, fish, dairy, legumes, tofu, and protein powders.
- **Healthy Fats**: Fats provide sustained energy, particularly for longer workouts, and help with nutrient absorption.
    - **Sources**: Avocado, nuts, seeds, olive oil, and fatty fish like salmon.
- **Complex Carbohydrates**: Carbs are the body's primary energy source, fueling muscles and helping to maintain stamina.
    - **Sources**: Whole grains, sweet potatoes, oats, and fruits.
- **Micronutrients**:
    - **Calcium and Magnesium**: Essential for muscle contractions and recovery. These minerals help prevent cramps and support muscle relaxation after intense workouts.
        - **Sources**: Leafy greens, nuts, seeds, and dairy products.

o **Vitamin D**: Supports bone health, which is crucial for lower body stability and strength.
  - **Sources**: Sunlight exposure, fortified foods, and supplements.

This section outlines the importance of these nutrients, along with suggested foods for each category, to help readers build a nutrient-dense diet that supports their fitness goals.

Hydration for Performance and Recovery

Hydration is essential for muscle performance, endurance, and recovery. Dehydration can lead to muscle fatigue, cramps, and hindered performance, which is why it's crucial to stay hydrated before, during, and after workouts.

- **Pre-Workout Hydration**: Start the workout well-hydrated by drinking water throughout the day. Aim for 16-20 ounces 1-2 hours before exercising.
- **During Workout**: Drink small sips of water, especially during intense or long workouts, to maintain hydration.
- **Post-Workout**: Replace lost fluids by drinking 20-24 ounces for every pound of weight lost during exercise.

Readers are given tips on tracking hydration, such as using water bottles with volume markers or flavoring water naturally to encourage consistent drinking throughout the day.

Sample Pre- and Post-Workout Meals and Snacks

To make nutrition practical and accessible, this section provides readers with easy meal and snack ideas that meet the nutritional needs of lower body workouts.

- **Pre-Workout Ideas**:
    o Greek yogurt with berries and honey
    o Whole-grain toast with almond butter and banana slices
    o A smoothie with oats, protein powder, and a handful of spinach
- **Post-Workout Ideas**:
    o Grilled chicken with quinoa and steamed vegetables
    o Cottage cheese with pineapple and a sprinkle of chia seeds
    o Protein shake blended with a banana and almond milk

By following these pre- and post-workout suggestions and incorporating the key nutrients outlined in this chapter, readers will be better equipped to fuel their workouts, enhance performance, and support their journey toward achieving toned, strong hips and thighs.

Protein for Muscle Repair and Growth: Supporting Strength and Definition

Protein is fundamental for repairing and building muscles, especially after strength training sessions that work the lower body. Muscles experience minor tears during exercise, and protein provides the amino acids needed to repair these fibers, allowing them to grow stronger and more defined.

- **Daily Protein Goals**: For muscle toning and growth, aim for around 0.7-1 gram of protein per pound of body weight. This range supports repair, helps prevent muscle loss, and promotes the growth of lean muscle in the hips, thighs, and glutes.
- **Easy Meal Ideas to Hit Daily Protein Targets**:
  - **Breakfast**: Greek yogurt parfait with berries, almonds, and a sprinkle of chia seeds.
  - **Lunch**: Quinoa salad with grilled chicken, mixed greens, and chickpeas.
  - **Dinner**: Salmon with roasted sweet potatoes and a side of steamed asparagus.
  - **Snacks**: Cottage cheese with pineapple, a handful of nuts, or a

protein shake with almond milk and a banana.

Including a protein source in each meal helps you meet your daily goals while keeping you energized and supporting post-workout recovery.

Anti-Inflammatory Foods for Joint Health: Reducing Soreness and Supporting Longevity

Since hip and thigh exercises often engage large muscle groups, maintaining joint health is crucial for long-term fitness and mobility. Consuming anti-inflammatory foods can help reduce post-workout soreness and prevent joint issues that may arise with intense training.

- **Key Anti-Inflammatory Foods**:
  - **Fatty Fish** (such as salmon, mackerel, and sardines): Rich in omega-3 fatty acids, which reduce inflammation in muscles and joints.
  - **Leafy Greens** (like spinach and kale): High in antioxidants and vitamins that protect cells from inflammation.
  - **Berries** (blueberries, strawberries, etc.): Contain polyphenols and vitamin C that combat oxidative stress.

- o **Nuts and Seeds** (almonds, chia seeds, and walnuts): Provide omega-3s and fiber, both of which help reduce inflammation.
  - o **Turmeric and Ginger**: Known for their anti-inflammatory properties, these spices can be added to meals or smoothies.
- **Meal Ideas for Joint Health**:
  - o **Breakfast**: Oatmeal with a sprinkle of chia seeds, blueberries, and a dash of turmeric.
  - o **Lunch**: Spinach salad with walnuts, grilled salmon, and a lemon-turmeric vinaigrette.
  - o **Dinner**: Stir-fried veggies with ginger and a serving of brown rice and tofu.
  - o **Snacks**: A handful of almonds or a smoothie with spinach, berries, and a small piece of fresh ginger.

Incorporating these foods into your diet can support joint health and reduce inflammation, helping you recover faster and perform at your best. With a balance of protein for muscle growth and anti-inflammatory foods for joint health, you'll be set up for both strength gains and long-term lower body wellness.

By focusing on these nutritional pillars, readers will find it easier to achieve their goals of building strong, toned hips and thighs, while also supporting joint health and overall recovery for sustainable fitness progress.

Chapter 13: Essential Stretches for Hips and Thighs

Stretching is a vital part of any lower body workout routine, as it helps improve flexibility, reduce muscle tension, and prevent injury. This chapter provides a comprehensive guide to stretching exercises specifically targeting the hips and thighs, with routines to warm up your muscles and cool down effectively. By incorporating these stretches, you can enhance your performance, support muscle recovery, and promote long-term joint health.

Dynamic Warm-Up Stretches: Preparing Muscles for Strength Training

Dynamic stretching uses movement-based stretches to prepare the muscles and joints for the demands of a workout. These warm-up exercises are designed to increase blood flow, enhance your range of motion, and prime the hips and thighs for the exercises ahead.

- **Leg Swings**: Stand next to a wall or support. Swing one leg forward and back in a controlled motion, keeping the core engaged. This movement targets the hip flexors, hamstrings, and glutes, warming up the lower body.
    - **Sets and Reps**: Perform 10–15 swings on each leg.

- **Walking Lunges with a Twist**: Step forward with one foot into a lunge position, lowering your back knee toward the ground. Twist your torso over the front leg to stretch the hip flexors, glutes, and quadriceps.
  - **Sets and Reps**: 10 lunges per side.
- **Hip Circles**: Stand with feet hip-width apart and hands on hips. Make large, circular movements with your hips, alternating directions. This movement helps warm up the hip joint and activate stabilizing muscles.
  - **Sets and Reps**: 10 circles in each direction.
- **Knee Hugs**: Stand tall and lift one knee to your chest, hugging it with both arms and gently pulling it closer. Alternate legs to engage and stretch the hip flexors, glutes, and hamstrings.
  - **Sets and Reps**: 10 hugs per side.

Dynamic stretches like these prime the lower body for a full range of movement, improving workout performance and reducing the risk of strains or injuries.

Cool-Down Stretches: Flexibility, Recovery, and Relaxation

Cooling down after a workout with static stretching helps to relax the muscles, reduce soreness, and prevent tightness in the hips and thighs. These stretches focus on lengthening the muscles you've worked, promoting flexibility and aiding in recovery.

- **Seated Forward Fold**: Sit on the ground with legs extended forward. Slowly reach for your toes, bending at the hips. This stretch targets the hamstrings, calves, and lower back, releasing tension after intense lower body exercises.
    - **Hold**: 20–30 seconds, breathing deeply.
- **Figure Four Stretch**: Lie on your back, cross one ankle over the opposite knee, and gently pull the uncrossed leg toward your chest. This stretch is excellent for the glutes and outer hip muscles.
    - **Hold**: 20–30 seconds per side.
- **Butterfly Stretch**: Sit with the soles of your feet together, allowing your knees to fall outward. Gently press your knees down with your elbows, leaning forward to deepen the stretch in the inner thighs and groin.
    - **Hold**: 20–30 seconds.
- **Lying Quad Stretch**: Lie on your side and grab the top of one foot, pulling it gently toward your glutes. This position stretches the quadriceps, alleviating tension in the front of the thigh.
    - **Hold**: 20–30 seconds per side.
- **Hip Flexor Stretch**: Kneel with one knee on the floor and the other leg forward,

creating a 90-degree angle with both legs. Shift your weight forward slightly, stretching the hip flexor of the back leg. This stretch counteracts tightness from lower body exercises and sitting.

- o **Hold**: 20–30 seconds per side.

Regularly performing these cool-down stretches after workouts will help improve flexibility, enhance muscle recovery, and reduce the risk of injury.

By combining dynamic warm-ups with thorough cool-down stretches, you can optimize each workout for both immediate performance and long-term results. This focus on flexibility and recovery will help readers move forward in their fitness journey with a strong, mobile, and resilient lower body.

Hip and Thigh Mobility Drills: Maintaining Flexibility and Supporting Movement Quality

Mobility drills for the hips and thighs are essential for enhancing the body's ability to move freely and efficiently. These exercises focus on maintaining flexibility, improving range of motion, and supporting proper alignment, which are vital for lower body workouts and everyday activities. Including these mobility drills regularly in your routine can reduce stiffness, improve posture, and prevent injuries by ensuring your muscles and joints work harmoniously.

Here are some of the most effective hip and thigh mobility exercises, which are easy to incorporate into your warm-up or cool-down routines.

- **90/90 Hip Stretch**: Sit on the floor with one leg in front of you, bent at 90 degrees, and the other leg behind you, also bent at 90 degrees. Keep your torso tall and gently lean forward over the front leg to deepen the stretch. This move opens up the hip joints and engages deep hip rotators.
    - **Hold and Repeat**: 20–30 seconds on each side, repeating 2–3 times.
- **Deep Squat Hold**: Stand with feet slightly wider than shoulder-width apart and squat down as low as you can, keeping your chest up and weight on your heels. Hold the position and gently shift your weight side to side, which stretches the hips, thighs, and glutes while improving squat depth.
    - **Hold and Repeat**: 20–30 seconds, shifting weight for added range of motion.
- **Hip CARs (Controlled Articular Rotations)**: Stand on one leg or hold onto a support. Lift the opposite knee up, then rotate it out to the side, keeping the movement controlled and slow. Rotate the knee back and down to the starting

position. This exercise increases hip mobility by working through the full range of motion.

  - o **Sets and Reps**: 5–10 controlled rotations per side.
- **Cossack Squat**: Stand with feet wide apart. Shift your weight onto one leg, bending that knee while keeping the opposite leg straight. Sink down as far as you can, stretching the inner thigh of the straight leg. Switch sides and repeat. Cossack squats are excellent for lateral mobility and flexibility in the hips and inner thighs.
  - o **Sets and Reps**: 5–10 reps on each side.
- **Lizard Pose**: Step one foot forward into a lunge position with your hands on the ground inside the front foot. Drop your back knee if needed, and allow your hips to sink down. This deep stretch targets the hip flexors, glutes, and inner thighs, releasing tightness and promoting flexibility.
  - o **Hold**: 20–30 seconds per side, taking deep breaths.
- **Leg Circles (Supine)**: Lie on your back with one leg straight up toward the ceiling. Make small to medium-sized circles with the raised leg, keeping your core engaged. This exercise gently mobilizes the hip joint, promoting stability and flexibility.
  - o **Sets and Reps**: 10–15 circles per leg, in both clockwise and counterclockwise directions.

Benefits of Hip and Thigh Mobility Drills

Regularly incorporating mobility drills enhances flexibility, reduces muscle imbalances, and promotes a full range of motion, making lower body exercises safer and more effective. These exercises not only help reduce injury risk but also contribute to improved posture, reduced stiffness, and greater movement efficiency in everyday life. By prioritizing mobility, you'll enjoy stronger, more fluid movements that support both fitness goals and general well-being.

Chapter 14: Recovery Techniques and Injury Prevention

After putting in the hard work during your lower body workouts, it's equally important to focus on recovery and injury prevention. This chapter provides the essential techniques to help your muscles repair, grow stronger, and prevent injuries, ensuring that you can continue progressing toward your fitness goals without setbacks. Effective recovery practices are vital for long-term results and injury-free training.

Foam Rolling and Self-Massage: Techniques to Relieve Muscle Tension and Prevent Soreness

Foam rolling and self-massage are powerful recovery tools that help to alleviate muscle tension, reduce soreness, and improve flexibility. These techniques target muscle knots, release fascia (the connective tissue surrounding muscles), and enhance blood circulation, speeding up recovery and reducing the likelihood of injury. Here's how to perform these techniques effectively:

1. **Foam Rolling the Quadriceps**:
    - **How to Do It**: Lie face down with the foam roller placed under your thighs. Rest your upper body on your forearms for support and roll slowly

from your hips to your knees, targeting any tight spots.

- o **Duration**: Spend 1–2 minutes rolling each quadriceps. Pause on any tight areas for 20–30 seconds to release the tension.

2. **Foam Rolling the Hamstrings**:
   - o **How to Do It**: Sit on the ground with one leg extended and place the foam roller under your hamstring. Lift your hips off the ground and roll from your glutes to the back of your knee, focusing on any tight spots.
   - o **Duration**: Roll each hamstring for 1–2 minutes, paying attention to knots or tight areas.

3. **Foam Rolling the IT Band (Outer Thigh)**:
   - o **How to Do It**: Lie on your side with the foam roller placed under your outer thigh (starting from the hip and rolling down towards the knee). Use your upper body and opposite leg for support as you gently roll over the IT band.
   - o **Duration**: 1–2 minutes on each side. Stop and hold on any particularly tight spots for 20–30 seconds.

4. **Foam Rolling the Glutes and Lower Back**:
   - o **How to Do It**: Sit on the foam roller and cross one ankle over the opposite knee (figure-four position) to target

the glute muscles. Roll gently over the glute and lower back area, applying more pressure on areas of tension.

- o **Duration**: 1–2 minutes for each side.

5. **Self-Massage with a Massage Ball**:
   - o **How to Do It**: Using a massage ball (or tennis ball), place it on areas of muscle tension, like the glutes, calves, or shoulders. Roll the ball over the affected area, applying pressure to break up knots and improve blood flow.
   - o **Duration**: Hold for 30–60 seconds on tight spots, moving the ball gently over the muscles.

Signs of Overtraining: Recognizing Overuse and Preventing Common Lower Body Injuries

Overtraining is a common pitfall for individuals who push themselves too hard without adequate rest or recovery. It can lead to injuries, burnout, and plateauing in progress. Understanding the signs of overtraining and knowing how to prevent injuries are essential for maintaining consistent results while staying injury-free.

1. **Physical Signs of Overtraining:**

- **Persistent Muscle Soreness**: If you're constantly sore after workouts and this soreness doesn't improve after rest days, it may be a sign that your muscles haven't recovered properly.
- **Decreased Performance**: A sudden drop in strength, endurance, or overall performance despite regular training can indicate overtraining.
- **Fatigue**: Feeling constantly tired, sluggish, or lacking energy, even after a good night's sleep, is a red flag that your body is not recovering.
- **Sleep Disturbances**: Overtraining can disrupt sleep patterns, leading to difficulty falling or staying asleep. Poor quality sleep negatively impacts muscle recovery.
- **Increased Resting Heart Rate**: An elevated resting heart rate, especially upon waking, may indicate that your body is under stress and not fully recovered.

2. **Psychological Signs of Overtraining**:
   - **Irritability or Mood Swings**: Overtraining can lead to hormonal imbalances that affect mood, causing irritability, anxiety, or depression.
   - **Loss of Motivation**: A sudden loss of enthusiasm for working out or feelings of dread before your

workouts can be signs that your body is physically and mentally fatigued.

3. **Injury Prevention Tips**:
    o **Listen to Your Body**: Pay attention to pain, discomfort, or fatigue. If you experience sharp pain during an exercise, stop immediately and seek medical attention if necessary. Learn to distinguish between discomfort (normal muscle fatigue) and actual pain (which can indicate injury).
    o **Include Rest Days**: Rest is critical for muscle recovery and growth. Avoid training the same muscle group on consecutive days to allow muscles to repair and rebuild. Aim for at least 1–2 rest days per week.
    o **Warm-Up Properly**: Never skip your warm-up. It prepares your muscles and joints for more intense activity, reducing the risk of strains and sprains.
    o **Focus on Mobility and Flexibility**: Incorporate regular stretching and mobility work into your routine. Tight muscles are more prone to injury, especially in the hips, thighs, and glutes, which bear much of the workout load.
    o **Gradually Increase Intensity**: Avoid making drastic increases in weight, reps, or intensity. Progress gradually over time to prevent

overuse injuries, and track your improvements.

- o **Cross-Training**: Vary your workouts to avoid overuse of the same muscle groups. Incorporate different forms of exercise such as swimming, cycling, yoga, or pilates to reduce the stress placed on your lower body.

4. **Common Lower Body Injuries and Prevention**:
    - o **Patellar Tendinitis (Runner's Knee)**: Often caused by overuse or improper movement patterns. Prevent this by strengthening the quadriceps, hamstrings, and glutes and avoiding excessive impact.
    - o **Iliotibial (IT) Band Syndrome**: Caused by repetitive motion, particularly from running or squatting. Prevent this by foam rolling and stretching the IT band regularly and incorporating strengthening exercises for the hips and thighs.
    - o **Hamstring Strains**: Tight hamstrings are more susceptible to injury. Perform regular stretching and mobility exercises to improve flexibility and avoid muscle strains.
    - o **Hip Flexor Strains**: Overworking the hip flexors without proper stretching can lead to strains. Include stretches such as the hip flexor

stretch and lunges to improve flexibility.

Sleep and Recovery: The Critical Role of Rest and Sleep in Muscle Repair, Energy Levels, and Fitness Progress

Sleep is often overlooked in fitness routines, but it is a cornerstone of any successful workout regimen. Your muscles need time to repair and grow, and rest is when this process happens. Without proper sleep and recovery, the benefits of your hard work at the gym can be severely compromised. This section explores the critical role of sleep and rest in muscle repair, overall energy levels, and long-term fitness progress.

1. Muscle Repair and Growth During Sleep

When you engage in strength training or any high-intensity workout, your muscles undergo micro-tears. These micro-tears are a natural part of the muscle-building process, but they need time to heal. Sleep provides the perfect environment for this repair. During deep sleep, the body secretes growth hormone, which is essential for tissue growth and repair. This process is when muscle fibers rebuild, becoming stronger and more resilient.

- **The Role of Deep Sleep**: Deep sleep, or slow-wave sleep, is particularly important for muscle recovery. It is during this phase that the body undergoes the most significant repair processes. If you consistently miss out on deep sleep, you are hindering muscle recovery and growth.

- **Impact on Protein Synthesis**: Sleep is also a key time for protein synthesis—the process by which your body builds new proteins. These proteins are crucial for muscle recovery. If you skimp on sleep, your body's ability to synthesize proteins decreases, which can lead to slower recovery times and reduced muscle gains.

2. Energy Levels and Performance

Quality sleep plays an essential role in maintaining high energy levels throughout the day. When you get sufficient rest, your body is well-equipped to handle the physical demands of exercise and everyday activities. Poor sleep, on the other hand, can lead to fatigue, which directly impacts your workout performance.

- **Performance Decline**: Sleep deprivation can result in decreased strength, endurance, and coordination during workouts. You may feel sluggish, unmotivated, or even experience a decline in the quality of your workouts. Without rest, your body cannot fully recover from previous training sessions, leaving you vulnerable to fatigue and burnout.
- **Mental Focus**: Sleep isn't just important for physical recovery—it's vital for mental clarity and focus as well. When you are

well-rested, you're more likely to maintain proper form, follow through with your workouts, and push yourself to new limits. Sleep enhances cognitive function, helping you stay focused and energized throughout your training.

3. Hormonal Regulation

Sleep has a profound effect on the balance of hormones in your body, including those responsible for muscle recovery and fat loss.

- **Testosterone Levels**: Testosterone plays a key role in muscle growth and fat loss. Chronic sleep deprivation can lead to lower testosterone levels, which can negatively affect your muscle-building efforts. A good night's sleep helps maintain healthy testosterone levels, supporting strength training progress.
- **Cortisol and Stress**: Cortisol is a stress hormone that can break down muscle tissue when levels remain elevated for prolonged periods. Lack of sleep increases cortisol levels, leading to higher levels of stress on the body and impeding muscle recovery. Proper sleep helps regulate cortisol levels, ensuring that your body remains in an anabolic (muscle-building) state rather than a catabolic (muscle-breaking) one.

4. Sleep and Fat Loss

For those working on toning their hips, thighs, or any other body part, sleep can also play a crucial role in fat loss. During sleep, the body engages in repair processes that affect fat metabolism. Lack of sleep can impair insulin sensitivity and disrupt metabolic function, making it harder for the body to burn fat efficiently.

- **Leptin and Ghrelin**: Sleep also regulates two hormones that control appetite—leptin (which signals fullness) and ghrelin (which stimulates hunger). Poor sleep can lead to increased ghrelin and reduced leptin levels, causing increased hunger and cravings, which can hinder fat loss efforts.
- **Better Recovery Means Better Results**: The combination of improved hormonal balance, better recovery, and reduced stress will help you achieve better fat-burning results. When the body has sufficient rest, fat is more likely to be burned efficiently during physical activity and at rest.

5. Optimizing Sleep for Fitness Recovery

To maximize the benefits of sleep for muscle recovery and fitness progress, it's important to prioritize the quality of your rest. Here are some practical tips for optimizing your sleep for recovery:

- **Aim for 7–9 Hours of Sleep**: Adults should aim for 7 to 9 hours of sleep per night. While everyone's needs may vary slightly, most people find this amount of sleep supports optimal physical and mental recovery.
- **Create a Sleep-Friendly Environment**: Keep your bedroom cool, dark, and quiet. Limit exposure to screens (like phones, tablets, and computers) at least 30 minutes before bed to promote melatonin production, the hormone that helps you fall asleep.
- **Follow a Sleep Routine**: Establish a regular sleep schedule by going to bed and waking up at the same time each day. This helps regulate your circadian rhythm, making it easier to fall asleep and wake up feeling refreshed.
- **Avoid Stimulants**: Avoid consuming caffeine or heavy meals close to bedtime, as they can interfere with your ability to fall asleep.
- **Incorporate Relaxation Techniques**: Practices like meditation, deep breathing, or light stretching before bed can help reduce stress and prepare your body for a restful night's sleep.

Part 5: Staying Motivated and Achieving Lasting Results

Chapter 15: Staying Consistent for Long-Term Success

Building strong, toned hips and thighs takes time, dedication, and the right mindset. Consistency is key to achieving and maintaining results, as even the best workout routine will fall short without regular commitment. In this chapter, we'll focus on actionable strategies to help you stay motivated and consistent, ensuring that your hard work leads to lasting improvements in strength, shape, and confidence.

Setting Milestones: Achieving Progress with Realistic Goals

Setting both short- and long-term goals is essential to staying on track. Having clear milestones gives you specific targets to aim for, allowing you to measure progress over time and celebrate each step forward. Here's how to set achievable goals and stay motivated along the way.

- **Start with SMART Goals**: Begin by making your goals SMART (Specific, Measurable, Achievable, Relevant, Time-bound). For example, instead of a vague goal like "I want to get stronger," you could set a SMART goal like, "I want to increase the weight of my squat by 10 pounds within the next two months." This kind of goal is clear, trackable, and gives you a specific timeline to work within.

- **Break Down Long-Term Goals**: Large goals can feel overwhelming, so it's helpful to break them down into smaller, manageable steps. If your long-term goal is to achieve a certain level of lower body strength or appearance, set monthly or even weekly targets to focus on. Celebrate hitting each smaller milestone, as each one brings you closer to your ultimate goal.
- **Create Appearance and Strength-Based Goals**: A balanced approach to goal-setting involves combining appearance-based goals with functional, strength-oriented ones. For example, if your goal is to achieve more defined thighs, consider setting a complementary strength goal, like being able to do 15 full bodyweight squats with proper form or increasing the resistance on a leg press machine. This mix of goals ensures you're not only improving appearance but also gaining strength and functionality.

Tracking Progress: Seeing Your Growth Over Time

Tracking progress is an effective way to stay motivated, as it shows you concrete evidence of improvement. There are multiple ways to measure results, allowing you to pick the ones that resonate most with you.

- **Use Photos and Measurements**: Documenting your journey visually and numerically can be incredibly motivating. Take photos every four to six weeks and track measurements of your thighs, hips, and other key areas. This approach helps you notice changes in muscle tone, definition, and size that may not be visible from day to day.
- **Workout Logs**: Keeping a workout log is another way to track your progress and identify areas of improvement. Record the weights, reps, and sets for each exercise you perform, noting how you feel during each session. A workout log allows you to see gains in strength over time, and it's also a great tool for spotting patterns in your performance.
- **Strength Tests**: Perform a simple strength test every few months to gauge your improvement. Examples include timing how long you can hold a wall sit, tracking how many lunges you can do in one minute, or measuring your progress in weighted exercises like squats. These tests

give you tangible metrics to evaluate your fitness journey and highlight areas where you're excelling.

Creating a Support System: Accountability and Encouragement

A support system can make all the difference in staying committed. Whether it's a friend, family member, workout buddy, or online community, having someone to share your goals and progress with can provide valuable encouragement.

- **Workout Buddy**: Partnering with someone who shares similar fitness goals can make workouts more enjoyable and hold you accountable. On days when motivation is low, a workout buddy can encourage you to show up and put in the effort.
- **Join a Community**: Online fitness groups or classes can be a great way to connect with like-minded individuals. Many people find motivation through community challenges, where members share daily workouts, motivational posts, or progress photos. This shared experience can help keep you committed over the long term.
- **Share Your Goals with Family or Friends**: Letting the people in your life know about your goals can create a support

network. Friends and family can provide positive reinforcement, celebrate your milestones, and even join you in your fitness journey.

Building Resilience: Overcoming Obstacles and Staying Focused

Consistency isn't always easy. There will be days when motivation wanes or life gets in the way. Building resilience allows you to push through these times and stay focused on your long-term goals.

- **Embrace Small Wins**: Recognize and celebrate every win, no matter how small. Achieving small goals—like completing a week of planned workouts or mastering a new exercise—keeps you motivated and reminds you of your progress.
- **Prepare for Setbacks**: Understand that setbacks are a normal part of any fitness journey. Injuries, busy schedules, and changes in motivation happen. The key is to view setbacks as temporary, and to stay adaptable. If you miss a workout or have an off week, focus on getting back on track rather than giving up entirely.
- **Mindset Matters**: Keeping a positive mindset is essential to staying consistent. Remind yourself why you started, focus on the benefits you've already gained, and

envision the results you're working toward. A positive mindset makes it easier to show up, even on days when motivation is lacking.

Celebrating Small Wins: Recognizing Progress at Every Stage

Celebrating small wins is crucial for maintaining motivation and keeping the journey enjoyable. It's easy to focus only on the end goal, but acknowledging progress—no matter how small—helps build momentum and reminds you of how far you've come. Whether it's lifting a slightly heavier weight, mastering a new exercise, or feeling a boost in energy, each small win brings you closer to your larger fitness goals.

- **Track Milestones**: Even incremental improvements, such as lifting five pounds more or completing an extra set, show progress. Note these wins in your workout log or journal to see how they accumulate over time.
- **Reward Yourself**: When you hit a milestone, reward yourself with something that reinforces your fitness goals. New workout gear, a relaxing recovery day, or even a celebratory meal can serve as a meaningful reminder of your hard work.
- **Reflect on Progress**: Every few weeks, look back on where you started. Comparing your current progress with your initial state

is a powerful reminder of the positive changes that consistency brings.

Strategies for Overcoming Plateaus: Keeping Your Progress Moving

Hitting a plateau is common in any fitness journey, as your body adapts to routines over time. When progress slows, adjusting your approach can help you break through and continue advancing toward your goals.

- **Change Your Workout Routine**: Switching exercises, altering the number of sets and reps, or adding variety like supersets or circuits can challenge your muscles in new ways, preventing adaptation and re-igniting progress.
- **Increase Intensity Gradually**: Gradually increasing weights, resistance, or intensity is essential for continued growth. Even a small increase, like adding 5–10% more weight or trying a higher-resistance band, can make a difference in muscle engagement and strength gains.
- **Focus on Form and Mind-Muscle Connection**: As you become familiar with exercises, revisit your form and work on enhancing the mind-muscle connection. Concentrate on contracting the targeted muscles, which can improve the quality of each movement and optimize results.

- **Adjust Rest and Recovery**: Sometimes a plateau occurs because your body needs more recovery time. Consider adding an extra rest day or incorporating activities like foam rolling, stretching, or yoga to support recovery.
- **Stay Patient and Persistent**: Plateaus are a natural part of progress. Remember that the most important thing is to stay consistent, keep challenging yourself, and trust the process. Adjusting your routine and staying positive will help you break through these periods and keep achieving results.

Celebrating each small success and knowing how to adapt through plateaus will not only keep your motivation strong but also help you reach your goals for a stronger, more sculpted lower body.

Chapter 16: Building Confidence Through Fitness

Achieving physical fitness is as much a mental journey as it is a physical one. Building strength and tone in your hips and thighs not only improves your body but also enhances your mindset, boosting self-confidence and self-belief. This chapter dives into the mental strategies and mindset shifts essential for staying motivated and patient as you work toward your goals, helping you cultivate a stronger, more positive outlook along the way.

Mindset Matters: Mental Strength for Physical Goals

A positive, resilient mindset is key to achieving lasting fitness results. Your approach to fitness should be as much about mental growth as it is about physical changes, as your mind will guide you through the most challenging moments and keep you moving forward when motivation fades.

- **Visualize Success**: Envisioning yourself achieving your goals is a powerful motivator. Whether it's lifting a heavier weight, completing a tough workout, or seeing the physical changes in your legs and hips, taking time to picture your success can help you push through difficult days.

- **Set Clear Intentions**: Begin each workout with an intention. Focus on what you want to accomplish in that session, such as pushing your limits, perfecting your form, or enjoying the movement. Clear intentions help turn each workout into a purposeful activity that builds confidence.
- **Stay Patient with Progress**: Fitness is a journey, and progress is often gradual. Patience helps you stay committed through the ups and downs. Instead of focusing solely on the end goal, appreciate the small, positive changes that happen over time. Patience allows you to enjoy the process and view each workout as a step forward, even if the changes seem slow.

Strategies for Staying Mentally Strong and Motivated

Motivation can fluctuate, but having strategies to keep your mind engaged and inspired will help you remain consistent.

- **Focus on Daily Wins**: Shift your focus from long-term results to what you can accomplish each day. Completing a workout, increasing reps, or feeling energized are all wins worth celebrating. When you focus on daily achievements, it keeps your confidence high and motivates you to keep going.

- **Embrace Setbacks as Learning Experiences**: Setbacks, whether due to injury, fatigue, or life's demands, are a normal part of the fitness journey. Instead of seeing setbacks as failures, view them as learning opportunities. Reflect on what happened, adjust your approach if needed, and come back stronger. This resilient mindset will keep you moving forward with confidence.

- **Cultivate Self-Compassion**: Many people are hard on themselves during their fitness journey, especially when progress is slower than expected. Being kind to yourself, acknowledging your efforts, and celebrating your persistence are essential for long-term success. Self-compassion reminds you that every effort counts, and that small steps add up to big results over time.

- **Practice Mindfulness**: Bringing mindfulness to your workouts helps you connect deeply with your body, making each movement more intentional. Pay attention to how your body feels as you perform each exercise, focus on your breathing, and be present in the moment. Mindfulness not only improves your workout quality but also builds a stronger connection between your mind and body, increasing your confidence as you see and feel progress.

How Fitness Builds Confidence Beyond the Gym

The confidence gained through fitness extends beyond physical appearance. The discipline, resilience, and self-belief you cultivate through your workouts shape your approach to other aspects of life as well.

- **Increased Body Awareness**: As you become more in tune with your body's abilities and limitations, your confidence naturally grows. Knowing that you can challenge yourself, push past limits, and accomplish physical feats helps you develop a more positive self-image and a deeper appreciation for your body.
- **Empowerment Through Physical Strength**: Physical strength and endurance translate into mental empowerment. When you see yourself capable of achieving physical goals, it reinforces your belief in your own strength and resilience in other areas of life, too.
- **Enhanced Self-Worth**: Fitness is a form of self-care, and by investing time in your health, you reinforce your own self-worth. Prioritizing fitness goals and sticking to them sends a powerful message to yourself that you are deserving of health, strength, and confidence.

Building confidence through fitness is a transformative journey that goes beyond aesthetics. As you grow stronger, both physically and mentally, you'll find a renewed sense of self-assurance, resilience, and self-love. This chapter will guide you in cultivating a mindset that supports long-term success, helps you navigate the challenges, and encourages you to celebrate the incredible progress you make along the way.

Body Image and Self-Acceptance: Fostering a Healthy, Positive Relationship with Your Body

Building strength, tone, and shape in your hips and thighs can certainly improve physical appearance, but one of the most profound transformations comes in the form of body image and self-acceptance. Learning to appreciate your body at every stage of your fitness journey not only helps you stay consistent but also fosters a healthier, more empowering relationship with yourself. This section explores strategies for cultivating self-acceptance and body positivity, creating a mindset that uplifts and motivates you no matter where you are in your journey.

---

1. Embrace the Process, Not Just the Outcome

Focusing on the process rather than an end goal allows you to appreciate every milestone along the way. Instead of seeing your body as a project to complete, view each workout, each stretch, and each moment of progress as a step in a lifelong journey of self-care and strength.

- **Shift Your Focus to Performance**: Track improvements in strength, endurance, and flexibility rather than just physical changes. Recognizing how your body becomes more capable over time builds a respect and appreciation for what it can accomplish, making physical transformations a bonus rather than the sole purpose.
- **Celebrate Non-Scale Victories**: Often, the most fulfilling milestones have nothing to do with appearance. Increased energy, improved sleep, reduced stress, and the ability to complete exercises you once found difficult are all victories that foster positive self-image.

2. Redefine What "Fit" Looks Like for You

Fitness is personal, and embracing your unique body shape and abilities is key to self-acceptance. Every body is different, and there's no single mold for what "fit" or "strong" should look like. By defining fitness in terms that resonate with your goals, needs, and preferences, you allow yourself to thrive in your own journey without comparing yourself to others.

- **Set Personalized Goals**: Focus on goals that align with your values, such as becoming stronger, feeling more energized, or achieving specific fitness milestones. This approach frees you from societal or aesthetic expectations and instead lets you celebrate the body you're actively working to strengthen and care for.
- **Reframe "Ideal" Images**: Rather than comparing your progress or body to images of others, reframe your ideal as the best, strongest, and healthiest version of yourself. This internal focus makes your fitness journey empowering and prevents the frustration that can come from unrealistic comparisons.

---

3. Practice Self-Compassion on Challenging Days

Fitness journeys are not linear, and there will be days when motivation wanes or progress feels slow. Practicing self-compassion on these days is crucial. Being kind to yourself, rather than critical, helps you move past setbacks without guilt or frustration.

- **Accept Imperfections**: Remember that every body has areas of perceived imperfection, and these do not define your worth. Embracing imperfections as part of what makes your body uniquely yours fosters a more positive and accepting outlook.

- **Reframe Negative Self-Talk**: Catch yourself when you feel critical thoughts emerging, and replace them with affirmations of what you're proud of, both physically and mentally. By practicing gratitude for your body and its abilities, you can shift from judgment to appreciation.

4. Appreciate Your Body at Every Stage

Whether you're just starting out or already seeing changes, embracing your body at each stage of your journey builds confidence and self-love. Your body is continually adapting and growing stronger, and respecting its capabilities fosters a lasting sense of pride and acceptance.

- **Document Progress Beyond Photos**: While visual progress can be motivating, don't let it be your only measure. Use workout journals to capture moments of accomplishment, jot down positive feelings after a tough workout, or note small milestones. These reminders of your journey help you celebrate your body for its functionality and resilience, not just appearance.
- **Be Present with Your Body**: Practicing mindfulness during workouts—focusing on your breath, the feel of muscles engaging,

and the grounding of your feet—allows you to connect with your body in a positive way. This appreciation of movement, rather than just outcomes, builds a sense of unity between mind and body.

5. Emphasize Long-Term Health and Wellness

Lastly, view your fitness journey as a long-term investment in your health, wellness, and happiness rather than a short-term fix. When you prioritize lasting health and functionality, the focus shifts from immediate physical results to sustaining a strong, healthy, and confident body for life.

- **Prioritize Function Over Aesthetics**: Strong, toned legs and hips are more than just an aesthetic goal—they support you in everyday activities, enhance mobility, and protect you from injuries. By seeing fitness as a pathway to health and independence, you build a lasting respect for what your body can achieve.
- **Value Yourself Beyond Appearance**: Remember that fitness is one aspect of who you are. Focusing on qualities like strength, determination, resilience, and self-discipline builds a self-image rooted in positivity and self-worth.

Building strong, toned hips and thighs is an empowering goal, but fostering a positive relationship with your body is even more transformative. By embracing self-acceptance, focusing on progress over perfection, and celebrating your body at every stage, you can cultivate confidence, pride, and a sustainable love for fitness that extends far beyond the mirror.

Inspiring a Lifelong Love of Movement: Cultivating Joy in Exercise for Physical and Mental Health

Finding joy in movement is a powerful, often overlooked aspect of fitness. When you learn to see exercise as a rewarding, enjoyable activity rather than just a means to an end, you're more likely to stay consistent, achieve results, and benefit from physical and mental health improvements for life. Embracing movement as something that enriches your well-being creates a positive relationship with fitness, turning it from a chore into a cherished habit.

1. Discovering the Physical Benefits Beyond Aesthetics

It's easy to focus on the external results of exercise, but the internal benefits—such as increased energy, endurance, and improved cardiovascular health—provide lasting motivation. The physical rewards of exercise go beyond appearance; they enhance your quality of life in ways that make movement feel worthwhile on a deeper level.

- **Increased Vitality**: Regular movement boosts energy, making daily tasks feel easier and increasing your stamina. Feeling capable and energized creates positive feedback, reinforcing a desire to move.
- **Health Benefits That Last**: Building strong hips and thighs not only shapes your body but also helps protect your joints, improve bone density, and support heart health. These health benefits contribute to a longer, healthier life and reinforce the habit of consistent movement.

2. The Mental Rewards of Exercise

Exercise has profound effects on mental well-being, and learning to associate movement with these mental benefits can make fitness a habit that enhances your entire lifestyle. From stress relief to improved mood, exercise becomes a powerful tool for mental health as much as for physical transformation.

- **Mood Boosting and Stress Relief**: Physical activity releases endorphins, reducing stress and improving mood.

Whether it's the sense of accomplishment after a tough workout or the meditative quality of steady movement, exercise becomes a source of mental clarity and positivity.

- **Increased Resilience**: The discipline and persistence cultivated through fitness carry over into other areas of life. Overcoming challenges, setting and achieving goals, and pushing past perceived limits all build a mindset of resilience and self-confidence.

---

3. Exploring Different Types of Movement

Movement is most enjoyable when you find activities that genuinely excite and challenge you. This book offers diverse exercises, routines, and approaches to lower body fitness so you can discover what you love. Trying new forms of movement keeps fitness interesting and sustainable, while also giving you a broader skill set.

- **Variety for Enjoyment**: Trying bodyweight exercises, kettlebell workouts, plyometrics, and resistance band routines can make fitness exciting and less monotonous. The variety also allows you to explore different styles, so you find movements that feel rewarding and engaging.

- **Discovering Personal Preferences**: When you find the types of exercise that suit you best, movement stops feeling like a duty and starts becoming a part of your routine that you genuinely look forward to. For example, some people thrive in high-intensity intervals, while others prefer the slower burn of strength workouts.

4. Building a Routine You Love

To cultivate a lifelong love of movement, consistency is key. Building a routine that you enjoy, look forward to, and can adapt as your life changes makes exercise sustainable. This book helps you create a routine tailored to your preferences, abilities, and goals, allowing fitness to naturally fit into your lifestyle.

- **Setting Realistic Goals**: Goals that feel achievable and exciting make it easier to stay committed. Instead of focusing solely on aesthetic changes, setting goals around strength, flexibility, or endurance encourages a holistic appreciation for the progress you're making.
- **Creating Routines Around Your Life**: Consistent movement doesn't need to be time-consuming or disruptive. The routines in this book can be customized to fit your schedule, with options for short, efficient

workouts that are easy to incorporate into even the busiest day.

---

5. Embracing Exercise as a Form of Self-Care

Exercise is a valuable tool for self-care, allowing you to dedicate time to yourself and focus on your well-being. Viewing fitness as a form of self-nourishment, rather than punishment, turns movement into a positive part of your routine that supports both your physical and mental health.

- **Movement as "You Time"**: Dedicating time for exercise gives you a chance to recharge, reflect, and reconnect with your body. This intentional time helps you develop a loving relationship with fitness, and the focus shifts from "I have to work out" to "I get to move my body."
- **A Celebration of What Your Body Can Do**: Over time, exercise becomes a celebration of your body's strength, resilience, and adaptability. Embracing this mindset of appreciation and gratitude makes movement feel fulfilling, further supporting a lifelong habit of regular fitness.

---

6. Making Movement Part of Your Identity

When fitness becomes an enjoyable and consistent part of your routine, it naturally integrates into your lifestyle and becomes part of who you are. Over time, movement becomes less about specific goals and more about the sense of balance, well-being, and joy it brings to your life.

- **Developing a Routine that Evolves with You**: A sustainable fitness journey is flexible. As you grow stronger or your interests change, you can modify your routines to keep challenging and inspiring you. This adaptability helps make fitness a permanent, enjoyable fixture in your life.
- **Long-Term Motivation and Rewards**: Seeing exercise as a lifelong journey opens the door to continuous growth, learning, and self-improvement. With each milestone, you build confidence, expand your capabilities, and reinforce a love for movement that becomes a lasting source of joy.

Inspiring a lifelong love of movement means building a fitness habit that goes beyond aesthetics or short-term goals. When exercise is rooted in joy, self-care, and personal fulfillment, it becomes a lasting source of empowerment that benefits both body and mind. This book is your guide to making lower body fitness a powerful, enjoyable, and lifelong pursuit that enhances every aspect of your health and well-being.

Conclusion: Your Journey to Stronger, Sculpted Legs

As you come to the end of this book, remember that building a strong, sculpted lower body is not just about achieving a visual goal; it's a journey of strength, resilience, and self-empowerment. Every step forward, every set completed, and every milestone reached adds up to meaningful progress that you can be proud of. Embrace this process, knowing that true fitness is a blend of persistence, self-compassion, and celebrating the small wins along the way.

The routines, exercises, and insights in this book are designed to guide you, offering the flexibility to grow with you as your strength and endurance improve. Take pride in each accomplishment, however small, and acknowledge the effort you're putting into this journey. Fitness is as much about the mental rewards as the physical ones—every workout you complete not only brings you closer to your physical goals but also builds confidence and resilience that extend far beyond the gym.

Remember, the benefits of a strong lower body are enduring. With healthy, toned, and powerful legs, you're setting the foundation for a more active, capable, and enjoyable life. These muscles support your posture, improve your balance, and protect you from injury, helping you move with grace and confidence through all that life brings.

As you move forward, let the tools in this book serve as a lasting resource. Whether you're just starting or you're looking to level up your routine, you now have a complete guide to support your lower body fitness journey. May this be a lifetime of healthy movement, inner strength, and a true love for all that fitness brings. Here's to strong, confident, and sculpted legs that carry you toward a more vibrant and fulfilling future.

www.ingramcontent.com/pod-product-compliance
Lightning Source LLC
Chambersburg PA
CBHW061036250726
48653CB00001B/122